Autologous Resurfacing and Fracture Dowelling

Klaus Draenert · Yvette Draenert
Tim Pohlemann · Gerd Regel

Autologous Resurfacing and Fracture Dowelling

A Manual of Transplantation Technique

Foreword by Allan E. Gross

In Collaboration with:
F. Baumgaertel, J. Bruns, M.E. Draenert, A.I. Draenert, F. Draijer, and M. Erler

with Clinical Support from:
R. Aufenberg, K. Blaesius, G. Bongaerts, E.-W. Braeuchle, K.E. Brinkman,
R. Chlebusch, U. Culemann, D. Daiber, St. David, H. Eckardt, J. Eulert,
A. Ekkernkamp, F. Fernandez, A. Friedrich, U. Garde, B. Gerber, U. Gras,
M. Gunselmann, C.-H. Hartwig, J. Hauert, St. Heinz, Th. Joka, W. Knopp,
E. Kollig, H. Kraemer, R. Labitzke, H.G. Laprell, U. Maronna, J. Mathé,
K.A. Matzen, H.-J. Michel, H.M. Mittag, J.-P. Mueller, D. Nast-Kolb,
M. Naupert, H.-D. Paschmeyer, G. Pattay, N. Pfannmueller, U. Quint,
J. Radke, M. Rischke, B. Rischke, St. Ruchholtz, M. Runkel, K. Russe,
A. Schneider, E. Schütz, P. Singewald, H.-W. Springorum, H.-U. Stäubli,
L. Tessari, B. Thomas, K. Ullrich, Ch. Ulrich, N. Walker, A. Wentzensen,
J.-P. Woltersdorf

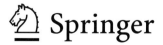

Authors

Prof. Dr. Klaus Draenert
Zentrum für Orthopädische
Wissenschaften
Gabriel-Max-Straße 3
81545 München
Germany

Prof. Dr. Tim Pohlemann
Universitätsklinikum des
Saarlandes
Klinik für Unfall-, Hand- und
Wiederherstellungschirurgie
Kirrberger Str.
66421 Homburg
Germany

Dr. Yvette Draenert
Zentrum für Orthopädische
Wissenschaften
Gabriel-Max-Straße 3
81545 München
Germany

Prof. Dr. Gerd Regel
Klinikum Rosenheim
Unfallchirurgie
Pettenkoferstraße 10
83022 Rosenheim
Germany

ISBN 978-3-642-24910-5   ISBN 978-3-642-24911-2 (eBook)
DOI 10.1007/978-3-642-24911-2
Springer Heidelberg Dordrecht London New York

Library of Congress Control Number: 2012933961

© Springer-Verlag Berlin Heidelberg 2012
This work is subject to copyright. All rights are reserved by the Publisher, whether the whole or part of the material is concerned, specifically the rights of translation, reprinting, reuse of illustrations, recitation, broadcasting, reproduction on microfilms or in any other physical way, and transmission or information storage and retrieval, electronic adaptation, computer software, or by similar or dissimilar methodology now known or hereafter developed. Exempted from this legal reservation are brief excerpts in connection with reviews or scholarly analysis or material supplied specifically for the purpose of being entered and executed on a computer system, for exclusive use by the purchaser of the work. Duplication of this publication or parts thereof is permitted only under the provisions of the Copyright Law of the Publisher's location, in its current version, and permission for use must always be obtained from Springer. Permissions for use may be obtained through RightsLink at the Copyright Clearance Center. Violations are liable to prosecution under the respective Copyright Law.
The use of general descriptive names, registered names, trademarks, service marks, etc. in this publication does not imply, even in the absence of a specific statement, that such names are exempt from the relevant protective laws and regulations and therefore free for general use.
While the advice and information in this book are believed to be true and accurate at the date of publication, neither the authors nor the editors nor the publisher can accept any legal responsibility for any errors or omissions that may be made. The publisher makes no warranty, express or implied, with respect to the material contained herein.

Illustrations: Reinhold Henkel, Heidelberg

Printed on acid-free paper

Springer is part of Springer Science+Business Media (www.springer.com)

Foreword

This manual introduces a surgical technique of bone and cartilage auto transplantation that has been perfected over many years by the authors. Prior to embarking on clinical material, the authors have many years of basic research on the anatomy, histology and growth of bone and cartilage. They have also experiments with ceramic bone substitutes and their use in reconstruction. They have perfected operative techniques using their innovative technology and their results, which I have witnessed personally, are extremely impressive, and hold promise for the future of this still young field of biological surgery.

The role of osteochondral transplantation for posttraumatic localized defects in young patients has been already established for the shoulder, elbow, knee and ankle. The authors expanded these techniques to include the wrist and the foot. The manual, which is superbly illustrated by drawings and case examples with x-rays and case intraoperative photos, is relatively straightforward. The contribution by the authors is of course in this technology they have invented and allows preservation of the cartilage when using these fine dowel techniques.

The first chapter deals with the history of bone and cartilage science. The history is interesting with many of the scientists whose names are familiar to us all being mentioned with reference to their contributions. There's an extensive bibliography and a collection of pictures and old articles that have been copied from the originals.

The next chapter is the microscopic anatomy of hyaline cartilage, epiphyseal cancellous bone and metaphyseal cancellous bone. The gross microscopic and electron microscopy pictures that are shown have all been produced out of the author's lab. The third and fourth chapters are related to bone growth and regeneration and healing of both cartilage and bone. These chapters are well referenced and illustrated with much of the work coming out of the author's lab.

It is important to note that the author's clinical expertise and surgical techniques were based on his own basic research conducted with his wife and colleagues in their laboratory, which is run completely by them.

The fifth chapter is related to the use of ceramics as bone substitutes. This once again is mainly a basic science chapter with a good bibliography, but some of the key articles and all of the illustrations once again based out of the Draenert lab.

After five chapters that deal with the basic science of bone and cartilage growth and repair, and the basic science of ceramic bone substitutes, the surgical manual starts with Chap. 6. The author's surgical technique for cartilage and bone transplantation is described in detail using the author's own surgical instrumentation developed in their laboratory. This chapter is beautifully illustrated with both drawings and photographs.

Chapter 7 deals with the clinical practice of autologous resurfacing in the knee, ankle and foot, hip and pelvis, shoulder, elbow, hand and wrist. Once again it is the authors' specific technique using their own surgical instrumentation. There are many case examples illustrating the surgical technique with the use of drawings and intraoperative photographs.

The eighth and ninth chapters deal with the author's technique for dealing with osteochondral fractures, non-unions and cruciate reconstruction.

The tenth chapter is a detailed description of the instrumentation. The eleventh chapter deals with the author's personal results of autologous resurfacing and fracture doweling, how to deal with donor areas and also their results with ceramics as bone substitute.

The authors have achieved excellent balance of basic research including anatomy and histology, and the gradual development of a special surgical technique, which thus far has produced outstanding results in the field of bone and cartilage transplantation.

Regards,

Allan E. Gross, MD, FRCSC

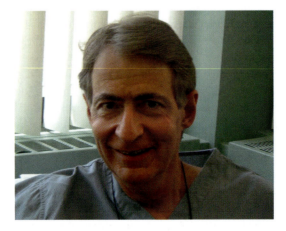

Preface

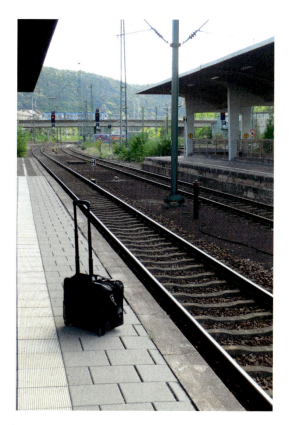

Stops along the way.....

The story began with a question regarding contact healing of single cancellous bone trabeculae. At the time, our first animal experiment using beagles was conducted under Hans Willenegger in Liestal in order to answer this gap of the ASIF (Association for the Studying of Internal Fixation) research group. It soon became clear that contact healing of single cancellous bone trabeculae was not possible applying compression osteosynthesis: Even when the cortical bones were in contact to each other, a space measuring 80 μm was still found between the cancellous trabeculae of our hemiosteotomy. Willenegger persisted and we also wanted to know the answer. The requirements were evident: the trabeculae on both sides had to be vital and undamaged. The only appropriate technique to achieve that goal was the wet-grinding procedure common in the histological laboratory, as well as a principle which could only be realized using extremely precise, self-guiding instruments. The development of such a set of precise grinding instruments, which fit together like twins, could remove the trabeculae cylinders, and could properly prepare a bed which would enable a stable press-fit anchorage, did not occur overnight. In close contact with Hans Willenegger, our path led us in the meantime to Maurice Mueller in Bern. Willenegger commented on the interim results:

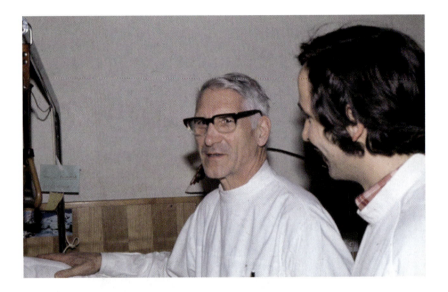

Dear Mr. Draenert,

Both volumes are an expression of your scientific engagement: the well-constructed experimental models which take a critical view of methodology, the later examinations, the outstanding staining procedures, and the fact that you still apply the 'thin-ground process'. This is how I remember you from your time in Liestal and this is how you have continued to develop.

Best wishes and greetings to you both,
H. Willenegger

Preface

Some of the twin instruments were developed in Bern, as were an entire series of experiments on rabbits, dogs and monkeys. Based on the results it was immediately clear: joint surgery would be changed forever. Maurice Mueller understood this at once. In the meantime, we moved to the Technical University of Munich, where, with the help of the DFG (German Research Council), we expanded our research in the Hospital Rechts der Isar.

Mueller and Willenegger continued supporting us financially, allowing the technology to step by step become reality. Maurice Mueller wrote in a visit to Munich:

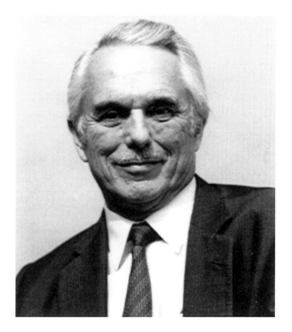

Leaving for Bern deeply impressed by the technical possibilities in the Draenert Institute and from the results achieved up until now.
Maurice Mueller

It took some time to obtain funding in Germany. The Ministry of Economic Affairs under Minister Wiesheu recognized the technology's future potential and promoted the completion of the entire instrument development within the framework of the Baytep program. We began to establish transplantation centers and to train in 2000. The period of travelling also began: rising early 146 times, waiting in train stations, taking off and landing in planes which crisscrossed the country, large BG hospitals, university hospitals as well as small private clinics. It was an exhausting but still fantastic time, operating with colleagues and convincing them that something should be done just so and no other way.

We made the difficult decision to end the initiative in 2002 in order to collect the results. We finally decided to call a meeting of users of the technology in Constance in 2006. The results were staggering: *restitutio ad integrum* in young patients with heavy necroses in the joint; full joint function in the case of the severest knee joint arthroses after 5 years, to name just a few examples. The path was open to us but the responsibility enormous because success depended and still depends on very precisely implemented and pre-planned reconstruction. Another intensive time of travel followed which focussed on the consolidation on operative planning and operative responsibility. The clear goal at this point, however, was to attract the support of a large, responsible company; a task in which we succeeded. We were able to win over Dr.h.c.mult. Sybill Storz and her son Karl-Christian to the value of our '*one step back to biology*'. The newly founded Recon Division of the Karl Storz GmbH & Co. KG in Tuttlingen has undertaken the objective of perfecting the *Diamond TwinS®* technology and introducing it onto the international market.

Prof. Dr. Klaus Draenert,
Dr. Yvette Draenert

Contents

1 Historical Observations 1
   1.1   Articulations 1
   1.2   Hyaline Cartilage 2
   1.3   Metaphyseal and Epiphyseal Bone 3
   1.4   Bone Growth 4
   References 11

2 Microscopical Anatomy 13
   2.1   Hyaline Cartilage 13
   2.2   Epiphyseal Cancellous Bone 15
   2.3   Metaphyseal Cancellous Bone 17
   References 20

3 Bone Growth 21
   3.1   Epiphyseal Growth 21
   3.2   Metaphyseal Growth 22
   3.3   Diaphyseal Growth 24
   References 27

4 Regeneration and Healing 29
   4.1   Hyaline Cartilage 29
   4.2   Epiphyseal Bone 31
   4.3   Metaphyseal Bone 32
   References 36

5 Ceramic Bone Substitutes 41
   5.1   Bioglasses 41
   5.2   Ceramics 41
      5.2.1   Bovine Ceramics 41
      5.2.2   Coralliform Ceramics 42
      5.2.3   Synthetic Ceramics – HA and ß-TCP 42
   5.3   Chemistry of Calcium Phosphates 43
   5.4   Osseoconduction – Bony Ingrowth 45
   5.5   Biodegradation 46
   5.6   Granulated Material 48
   References 51

6 Operating Technique for Cartilage-Bone Grafting 53
   6.1   Basic Principles 53
      6.1.1   Basic Guide to Instruments 53
      6.1.2   Diamond Twins 55

		6.1.3	Irrigation.	55
		6.1.4	Instrumentation Table.	56
		6.1.5	Cleaning of the Diamond Crowns	56
	6.2	Basic Steps of the Operating Technique		57
		6.2.1	Reparation of a Cartilage-Bone Defect	57
		6.2.2	Cutting the Cartilage	58
		6.2.3	Reconstructing the Donor Bed.	62
		6.2.4	The Donor Side Morbidity of the Iliac Crest	63
		6.2.5	Reparation of a Severe Cartilage-Bone Defect	63
		6.2.6	Reparation of a Complete Condyle with Damaged Cartilage	65
		6.2.7	Reparation of an Osteochondral Fragment	67
		6.2.8	A Tribute to the History of Bone Dowels	67
		6.2.9	Osteocartilage Fractures.	68
	6.3	The Donor Bed.		71
	References			74
7	**Clinical Practice in Autologous Resurfacing®.**			**77**
	7.1	Knee.		77
		7.1.1	Trauma.	77
		7.1.2	Osteochondritis Dissecans	81
		7.1.3	Osteoarthritis	81
	7.2	Ankle Joint and Foot		87
		7.2.1	Trauma.	87
		7.2.2	Osteochondritis Dissecans (Talus).	87
	7.3	Hip and Pelvis		92
		7.3.1	Trauma.	92
		7.3.2	Heel-Strike Osteoarthritis.	94
	7.4	Shoulder.		100
	7.5	Elbow.		101
	7.6	Hand and Wrist		101
	References.			111
8	**Fracture Dowelling**			**113**
	8.1	Osteochondral Fractures		113
	8.2	Dowelling of Nonunions		113
	References.			120
9	**Bone–Tendon–Bone ACL Plastic**			**121**
10	**Instrumentation.**			**123**
	References.			130
11	**Conclusion**			**131**
	11.1 The Success of Autologous Resurfacing and Fracture Dowelling			131
	11.2 The Donor Areals and Defects.			131
	11.3 Osteoconduction by Ceramics			131
	References.			132
Subject Index				**135**
Author Index				**137**

Historical Observations

1.1 Articulations

For a long time, little attention has been paid to articulations. Andreas Vesalius (1514–1564) mentioned them in his work *De humani corporis fabrica* (1543), however, without any morphological or functional analysis. On the wood engravings produced in Titian's studio, bones received the most attention and articulations were presented in lesser detail (Fig. 1.1).

G. Fallopio (1523–1562) discovered the growth plate without being able to interpret its function. In his *Observationes Anatomicae* (1562), he described cartilage as well as articulation and he mentioned the "articulo femoris et coxae" and also the articulation between scapula and humerus: "quo humerus et scapula iuguntur"; however, he never analyzed his findings. It took nearly two further centuries until articulations were more closely examined. R. Nesbitt (1736) dedicated his work to the development of bone from cartilage and the cartilaginous epiphyses, published in his book "Human Osteogeny" (Fig. 1.2).

Over time, anatomists and surgeons increasingly realized immoveable and moveable connections between the bones. Surgeons such as W. Cheselden, chief surgeon of the Royal Hospital at Chelsea, were mainly occupied with editing anatomical textbooks.

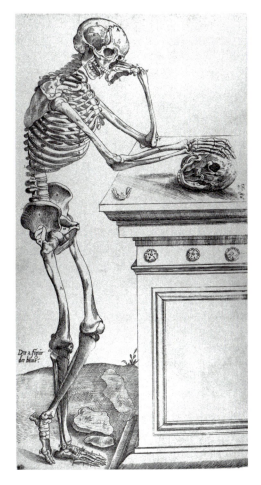

Fig. 1.1 Wood engravings from Titian's studio; the famous osteology and myology. "De humani corporis fabrica" of Andreas Vesalius (1555) Vesalius (1551)

K. Draenert et al., *Autologous Resurfacing and Fracture Dowelling*,
DOI 10.1007/978-3-642-24911-2_1, © Springer-Verlag Berlin Heidelberg 2012

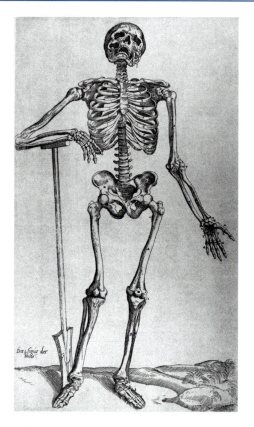

Fig. 1.1 (continued)

W. Cheselden (1756) had already described in detail the epiphyseal parts of long bones. He additionally classified the interarticular fibrocartilage, i.e., that of the temporomaxillary articulation, the menisci of the knee joint, as well as the ligaments of moveable joints. Cheselden wrote:

> Every part of a bone which is articulated to another bone for motion, is covered or lined with a cartilage, as far as it moves upon, or is moved upon by another bone in any action; for cartilage being smoother and softer than bone, it renders the motion more easy than it would have been, and prevents the bones wearing each other in their actions.

Cheselden had also already precisely described the menisci:

> In the joint of the knee are two loose, almost annular cartilages, which being thick at their outer edges, and thin at their inner ones, they make the greatest parts of the two sockets in this joint. The use of these cartilages is to make variable sockets to suit the different parts of the lower end of the os femoris.

Cheselden was the first to extract a biomechanical meaning from joint morphology and function and to present it in his work *The Anatomy of the Human Body* including 40 copperplate engravings (1756) (Fig. 1.3).

1.2 Hyaline Cartilage

In the beginning of the eighteenth century, surgeons and anatomists paid more attention to the hyaline articular cartilage. In 1743, the surgeon William Hunter, the elder brother of John Hunter, gave a detailed description of the hyaline cartilage. He founded the first private Anatomical Institute in London for obstetrics and gynecology.

The preciseness with which William Hunter at that time gave a detailed description of the hyaline cartilage, the joint, its capsule, and the ligaments' function is still remarkable. He wrote (Fig. 1.4). It was late, in the second half of the nineteenth century, that progress was made and more detailed studies on articular cartilage were published. Heidenhain (1863) stated that the cartilage cells were rounded and completely filled their sharply defined lacunae. Hammar (1894) published the first histomorphology of the hyaline cartilage. Hultkrantz (1897) had already determined the orientation of the collagen fibers with his "Spaltlinien" method, a milestone for all following discoveries. Schaffer (1897) defined the cell territory comprising the cell, capsule, and the interterritorial substance. Rathke introduced the term "cell-capsule." Based on the work of Hultkrantz, Benninghoff (1922) developed his functional morphology of the cartilage and defined the chondron as a functional unit. In 1925, he published his theory of the structure of hyaline cartilage, the course of fibers, their anchorage, and the reinforcement of the ground substance (Fig. 1.5a, b). A more detailed description followed later, again by Benninghoff (1939), who published the cell arrangement: a transitional zone containing oval or round cells following the tangential layer with flattened cells. This, in turn, follows a thicker, radial zone containing cell groups, which

1.3 Metaphyseal and Epiphyseal Bone

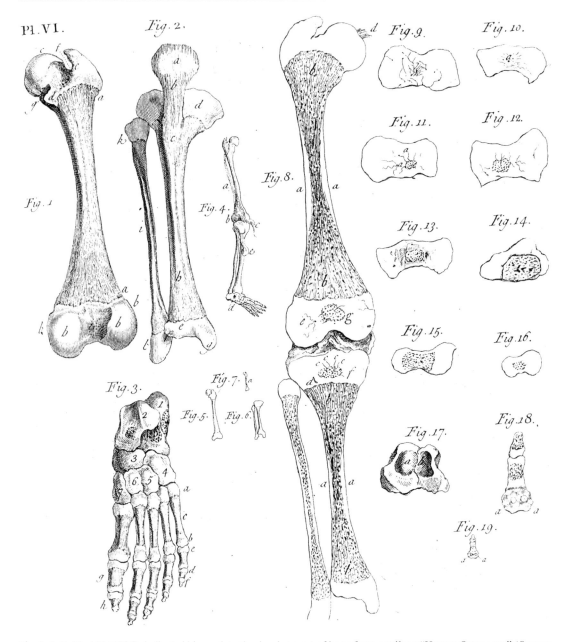

Fig. 1.2 R. Nesbitt (1736) dedicated his work to the development of bone from cartilage "Human Osteogeny" (*Source*: Nesbitt 1736, Pl. VI, Figs. 1–19)

is separated from the calcification zone by a wavy basophilic line.

Schmiedeberg (1891) defined chondroitin and chondroitin sulfate of the ground substance. Only MacConnail (1951) added his *lamina splendens*, a fiber-free layer on the surface of articular cartilage, to Benninghoff's description (1922, 1925, 1939).

1.3 Metaphyseal and Epiphyseal Bone

An anatomic description of the locomotor apparatus begins with Andreas Vesalius (1514–1564). His *Osteologia, Myologia and Cardiologia* was published on August 1, 1543, in Basel by Oporinus.

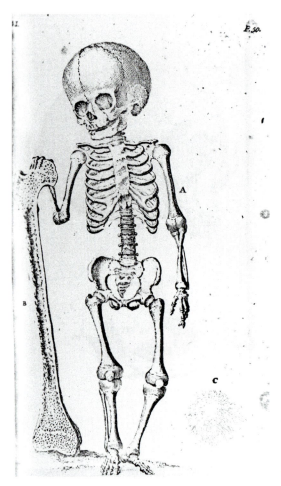

Fig. 1.3 W. Cheselden was first to describe the epiphyseal parts (**c**) of long bone (**a**, **b**) in detail (1756) (*Source*: Cheselden 1756, p. 50, Table II)

Biomechanics were first considered by Galileo Galilei (1638). He realized the importance of the biomechanical impact on bone morphology. More than a century later, Cheselden (1756) again mentioned the relationship between form and function, as well as between hollowness and bone strength. Hermann von Meyer (1867) described the trajectorial structuring of bone and analyzed the bone's morphology together with Culmann (1866). Finally, it was Julius Wolff (1892) who published his famous book based on that theory: *The Law of Transformation of Bones* (Fig. 1.6a, b). The Weber brothers from Wittenberg started the scientific analysis of the human gait and of the locomotor apparatus (Weber 1836).

Real progress was made with the work of William Harvey (1628). The circulation of the blood (*Exercitatio Anatomica de Motu Cordis et Sanguinis in animalibus*) was discovered. Anton van Leeuwenhoek's microscope was developed, and his observations of channels and pores in bone were published (1678). Clopton Havers reported in five lectures at the Royal Society of London (1691) on the structure and physiology of bone and recorded that in his *Osteologia Nova* in Latin with Georgium Wilhelmum Kühnium in Frankfurt (1692). The revised English edition *Some New Observations on Bone* (1731) (Fig. 1.7) and the corresponding edition in Latin (*Novae quaedam Observationes de Ossibus*, 1734) are today still considered classic contributions to bone research. Canals of Havers are first mentioned by Albinus (1757).

Leeuwenhoek (1678) had already reported the cell lacunae in the bony substance. Deutsch (1834) described "bony corpuscles" in the lacunae. Matthias Schleyden (1837) and Theodor Schwann (1839) had already published their cell doctrine. Based on that, Virchow (1850) identified those corpuscles as cell, which Koelliker (1867) named "Virchow's bone cells" and which in the published work of Weidenreich (1930) were called "osteocytes." Carl Gegenbaur (1864) introduced the term "osteoblasts" for the cells lining the bony surface which he regarded as the bone-forming cells. John Howship (1817) detected and described the surface lacunae, in which Robin (1864) described giant cells as "plaque à noyeau multiple." Lieberkühn (1861) defined the surface lacunae as "Howship's lacunae" and Koelliker (1872, 1873) proposed the term "osteoclast" for those giant cells. It was also Koelliker (1853, 1859) who named the ground substance "osteoid." Finally, Biedermann (1914) introduced the term "osteon" as a unit of bone constructions.

1.4 Bone Growth

The epiphyseal part of long bones (derived from the Greek "allow to grow") develops completely from cartilage (Nesbitt 1736). He had already

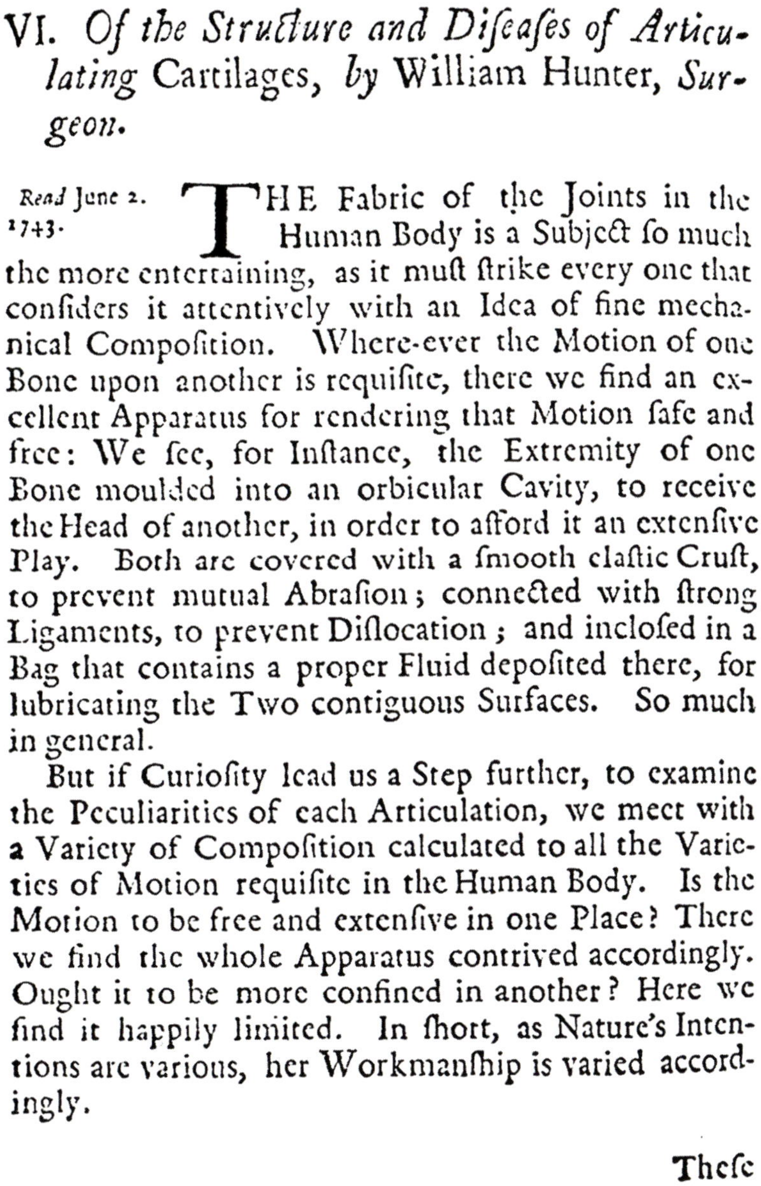

VI. *Of the Structure and Diseases of Articulating* Cartilages, *by* William Hunter, *Surgeon.*

Read June 2. 1743.

THE Fabric of the Joints in the Human Body is a Subject so much the more entertaining, as it must strike every one that considers it attentively with an Idea of fine mechanical Composition. Where-ever the Motion of one Bone upon another is requisite, there we find an excellent Apparatus for rendering that Motion safe and free: We see, for Instance, the Extremity of one Bone moulded into an orbicular Cavity, to receive the Head of another, in order to afford it an extensive Play. Both are covered with a smooth elastic Crust, to prevent mutual Abrasion; connected with strong Ligaments, to prevent Dislocation; and inclosed in a Bag that contains a proper Fluid deposited there, for lubricating the Two contiguous Surfaces. So much in general.

But if Curiosity lead us a Step further, to examine the Peculiarities of each Articulation, we meet with a Variety of Composition calculated to all the Varieties of Motion requisite in the Human Body. Is the Motion to be free and extensive in one Place? There we find the whole Apparatus contrived accordingly. Ought it to be more confined in another? Here we find it happily limited. In short, as Nature's Intentions are various, her Workmanship is varied accordingly.

These

Fig. 1.4 Lecture of William Hunter, the elderly brother of John Hunter, at the Royal Society of Biologists in London (1743) (*Source*: Hunter 1743)

These are obvious Reflections, and, perhaps, as old as the Inspection of dead Bodies. But modern Anatomists have gone further: They have brought the Articulations, as well as the other Parts of the Body, under a narrow Inquiry, and entered into the minutest Parts of their Composition. The Bones have been traced Fibre after Fibre; but the Cartilages, as far as I can learn, have not hitherto been sufficiently explained. After some fruitless Attempts by macerating and boiling the Cartilages in different *Menstrua*, I fell upon the Method not only of bringing their fibrous Texture to View, but of tracing the Direction and Arrangement of those Fibres. I shall therefore endeavour to give a short Account of the Structure of articulating Cartilages, and make a few Observations on their Diseases, with a View to advance a rational Explication of their morbid *Phænomena*.

An articulating Cartilage is an elastic Substance uniformly compact, of a white Colour, and somewhat diaphanous, having a smooth polished Surface covered with a Membrane; harder and more brittle than a Ligament, softer and more pliable than a Bone.

When an articulating Cartilage is well prepared, it feels soft, yields to the Touch, but restores itself to its former Equality of Surface when the Pressure is taken off. This Surface, when viewed through a Glass, appears like a Piece of Velvet. If we endeavour to peel the Cartilage off in *Lamellæ*, we find it impracticable; but, if we use a certain degree of Force, it separates from the Bone in small Parcels; and we never find the Edge of the remaining Part oblique, but always perpendicular to the subjacent Surface of the Bone. If we view this Edge through

Fig. 1.4 (continued)

a Glass, it appears like the Edge of Velvet; a Mass of short and nearly parallel Fibres rising from the Bone, and terminating at the external Surface of the Cartilage: And the Bone itself is planned out into small circular Dimples, where the little Bundles of the cartilaginous Fibres were fixed. Thus we may compare the Texture of a Cartilage to the Pile of Velvet, its Fibres rising up from the Bone, as the silky Threads of that rise from the woven Cloth or *Basis*. In both Substances the short Threads sink and bend in Waves upon being compressed; but, by the Power of Elasticity, recover their perpendicular Bearing, as soon as they are no longer subjected to a compressing Force. If another Comparison was necessary, we might instance the Flower of any corymbiferous Plant, where the *Flosculi* and *Stamina* represent the little Bundles of cartilaginous Fibres; and the *Calyx*, upon which they are planted, bears Analogy to the Bone.

Now these perpendicular Fibres make the greatest Part of the cartilaginous Substance; but without Doubt there are likewise transverse Fibrils which connect them, and make the Whole a solid Body, though these last are not easily seen, because being very tender, they are destroyed in preparing the Cartilage.

We are told by Anatomists, that Cartilages are covered with a Membrane named *Perichondrium*. If they mean the Cartilages of the Ribs, *Larynx*, Ear, *&c.* there, indeed, such a Membrane is very conspicuous; but the *Perichondrium* of the smooth articulating Cartilages is so fine, and firmly braced upon the Surface, that there is room to doubt whether

Fig. 1.4 (continued)

ther it has been often demonstrated, or rightly understood. This Membrane, however, I have raised in pretty large Pieces after macerating; and find it to be a Continuation of that fine, smooth Membrane that lines the capsular Ligament, folded over the End of the Bone from where that Ligament is inserted. On the Neck of the Bone, or between the Insertion of the Ligament, and Border of the Cartilage, it is very conspicuous, and may be pulled up with a Pair of Pincers; but where it covers the Cartilage, it coheres to it so closely, that it is not to be traced in the recent Subject without great Care and Delicacy. In this Particular it resembles that Membrane which is common to the Eye-lids and the Fore-part of the Eye-ball, and which is loosely connected with the *Albuginea*, but strongly attached to the *Cornea*.

From this Description it is plain, that every Joint is invested with a Membrane, which forms a complete Bag, and gives a Covering to every thing within the Articulation, in the same Manner as the *Peritonæum* invests not only the *Parietes*, but the Contents of the *Abdomen*.

Fig. 1.4 (continued)

discovered a connection between the epiphysis and the growth of long bones. It was H. Müller (1858), however, who made the interpretation of the so-called calcification and ossification nuclei. In the meantime, important experiments elucidated the secret of bone growth.

The rediscovery of the madder dye (Mizaldus 1566; Lemnius 1567) by London surgeon Belchier (1736) had an important impact on the subsequent experimental work on bone. Based on his experiments, Du Hamel (1739) started a series of experiments in which he also considered the discovery of the English clergyman Stephan Hales (1733), who had demonstrated with implanted bullets that bone grows at its ends – the part of bone which could be vitally stained. The series of Du Hamel was published in the *Histoire de l'Académie Royale des Sciences* (1741, 1742, 1743). According to his findings, only the newly formed bone could be labeled. Du Hamel became famous through his experiment with silver rings, with which he proved the growth in thickness by periosteal new bone formation: the silver rings tightly bound around the tube of the bone migrated through the cortex and were finally found in the medullary cavity (1742).

He defined the periosteum as "membrane ostéogène" and explained the growth by an interstitial growth of the bony tissue. The dialectic of bone apposition and simultaneous reabsorption was still unknown to him. It was John Hunter (1728–1793), the younger brother of William Hunter, who reached the breakthrough by repeating the experiments of Stephan Hales and H.L. Du Hamel. He managed to pass beyond the point at which both scientists had failed to make progress and had run into a dead-end. John Hunter articulated the basic principle of bone

1.4 Bone Growth

Fig. 1.5 (**a**, **b**) Benninghoff (1939) was the first to work out a detailed histomorphological analysis of the cartilage structure (*Source*: Benninghoff 1922)

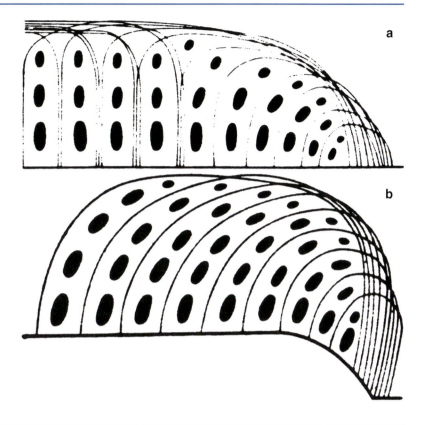

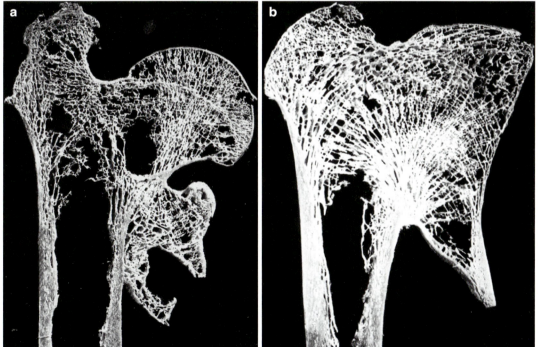

Fig. 1.6 (**a**, **b**) Samples of Julius Wolff, the German Surgeon from Berlin, who developed the theory of trajectories laid down in the Wolff's Law (1892) (*Source*: Wolff 1892, Figs. 1 and 2)

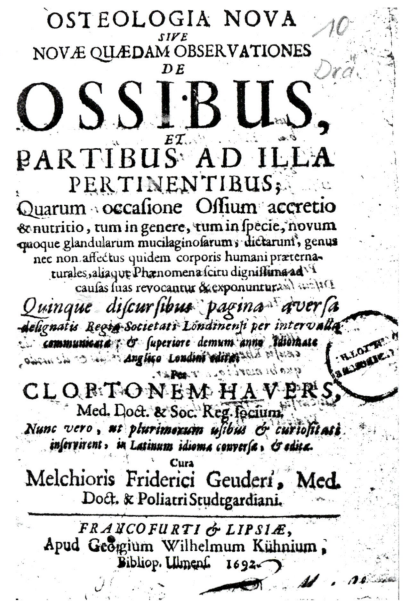

Fig. 1.7 The famous "Osteologia Nova" (1692) based on the published work of A. van Leeuwenhoek, who described "tubes and cylinders" in the bony substance (1678) in the "Philosophical Transactions" of the Royal Society of London (*Source*: Havers 1692)

growth, namely, that all bones grow by external apposition and inner simultaneous resorption. He also formulated the principle of bone turn over – "bone is constantly changing its matter" – and he died in 1793 believing that assumption without ever having had knowledge of the osteoclast. His "Experiments and Observations on the Growth of Bones" was published posthumously (1794, 1798).[1] Four decades later, Pierre-Jean Marie Flourens (1842, 1847) postulated that apposition and resorption are always combined processes remodeling the bony tissue. Hunter and Flourens were the discoverers of the bone remodeling process.

---

[1] The work of John Hunter was published in 1794 by Everard Home in the *Transactions of a Society for the Improvement of Medical and Chirurgical Knowledge* and later collected by James F. Palmer, together with his lectures since 1772, presented to the public in 1798, and edited as a book in 1835.

References

Albinus BS (1757) Academicarum Annotationum. Liber Septimus p 50. Verbeek, Leidae

Belchier J (1736) An account of the bones of animals being changed to a red colour by aliment only. Philos Trans R Soc Lond (Biol) 34:287–299

Benninghoff A (1922) Über den funktionellen Bau des Knorpels. Verh Anat Ges Erlangen 31:250–267

Benninghoff A (1925) Form und Bau des Gelenkknorpels in seinen Beziehungen zur Funktion. Z Zellforschg 2:763–862

Benninghoff A (1939) Lehrbuch der Anatomie des Menschen. Part I. Lehmann, München

Biedermann W (1914) Physiologie der Stütz- und Skeletsubstanzen. In: Winterstein (Hrsg) (ed) Handbuch der vergleichenden Physiologie 3, II.Teil. Gustav Fischer, Jena

Cheselden W (1756) The anatomy of the human body. Hitch and Dodsley, London

Culman K (1866) Die graphische Statik. Meyer und Zeller, Zürich

Deutsch C (1834) De penitiori ossium structura observationes. Inaug-Diss Vratislav, Breslau

Du Hamel HL (1739) Sur une racine qui a la faculté de teindre en rouge les os des animaux vivants. Mém de Mathématique et de Physique de l'Académie Royale des Sciences, Paris, pp 1–13

Du Hamel HL (1741) Observations sur la Réunion des Fractures des Os. Histoire de l'Académie Royale des Sciences. Imprimerie Royale, Paris, pp 97–112

Du Hamel HL (1742) Sur le Développement et la Crue des Os des Animaux. Histoire de l'Académie Royale des Sciences. Imprimerie Royale, Paris, pp 354–370

Du Hamel HL (1743) Mémoires sur les Os. Mem de l'Académie Royale des Sciences. Imprimerie Royale, Paris, pp 87–146

Fallopius G (1562) Observationes Anatomicae. Birkmann, Coloniae

Flourens P (1842) Recherches sur le Développement des Os et des Dents. Gide Libraire, Paris

Flourens P (1847) De la Formation des Os. JB Baillière, Paris

Galilei G (1638) Mechanik Dialog I Zitiert nach Evans FG (1957) Stress and strain in bones. ChC Thomas, Springfield

Gegenbaur C (1864) Über die Bildung des Knochengewebes. Jena Z Med Naturwiss 1:343–369

Hales S (1733) Haemastaticks. W and J Innys and T Woodward: London.

Hammar SA (1894) Über den feineren Bau der Gelenke. II.Abt. Der Gelenkknorpel. Arch Mikrosk Anat 43:813–885

Harvey GA (1628) Exercitatio anatomica de motu cordis et sanguinis in animali. Guilielmi Fitzeri, Francofurti

Havers C (1691) Osteologia nova (Phil Trans R Soc Lond 1689–1690). GW Kühnium, Francofurti

Havers C (1692) Osteologia Nova sive Novae Quaedam Observationes de Ossibus. GW Kühnium, Francofurti et Lipsiae

Havers C (1731) Some new observations on bone. GW Kühnium, Francofurti

Havers C (1734) Novae Quaedam Observationes de Ossibus. G Wishoff, Lugduni Batavorum (Leyden)

Heidenhain R (1863) Zur Kenntnis des hyalinen Knorpels. Stud Physiol Inst Breslau 21–31

Howship J (1817) Observations on the morbid structure of bones and attempt at an arrangement of their diseases. Med Chir Trans 8:57–107

Hultkrantz W (1897) Das Ellbogengelenk und seine Mechanik. Fischer, Jena

Hunter W (1743) Of the structures and diseases of articulating cartilage. Philos Trans R Soc Lond (Biol) 42: 514–521

Hunter J (1794) Experiments and observations on the growth of bones. In: Everard H (ed) Transactions of a society for the improvement of medical and chirurgical knowledge, vol II

Hunter J (1798) Experiments and observations on the growth of bones. In: Palmer JF (1835) (ed) The works of John Hunter FRS. Longman Rees Orme Brown Green and Longman, London, pp 315–318

Kölliker A (1853) Manual of human histology. In: Bush G (ed) 1:365. T. Huxley, Sydenham

Kölliker A (1859) Über verschiedene Typen in der mikroskopischen Struktur des Skelettes der Knochenfische. Verh physik-med Ges Würzburg 9

Kölliker A (1867) Handbuch der Gewebelehre des Menschen. 5. Auflage. W Engelmann, Leipzig

Kölliker A (1872) Die Verbreitung und Bedeutung der vielkernigen Zellen in Knochen und Zähnen. Verh physik-med Ges Würzburg 2:243

Kölliker A (1873) Die normale Resorption des Knochengewebes und ihre Bedeutung für die Entstehung der typischen Knochenformen. FCW Vogel, Leipzig

Lemnius L (1567) De miraculis occultis naturae. Colonia

Lieberkühn N (1861) Über den Abfall der Geweihe und seine Ähnlichkeit mit dem kariösen Prozess. Reichert's du Bois-Reymond's Arch 49:748–759

MacConaill MA (1951) Movements of bones and joints; mechanical structure of articulating cartilage. J Bone Joint Surg 33-B:251

Mizaldus A (1566) Memorabilium utilium et iucundorum centuriae. Lutetia

Müller H (1858) Über die Entwicklung der Knochensubstanz nebst Bemerkungen über den Bau rachitischer Knochen. Z Zool 9:147–233

Nesbitt R (1736) Human osteogeny. W Innys and R Manby, J Pemberton, E Symon, J Noon, and C Davis, London

Robin C (1864) Notes sur les éléments anatomiques appelés myéloplaques. J Anat Physiol Norm 1: 88–109

Schaffer J (1897) Die Verknöcherung des Unterkiefers und die Metaplasiefrage. Arch mikrosk Anat 32 IV

Schleyden MJ (1837) Beiträge zur Phytogenesis. Arch Anat wiss Med 137–176

Schmiedeberg O (1891) Über die chemische Zusammensetzung des Knorpels. Arch exper Path Pharmak 28

Schwann T (1839) Microscopical researches into the accordance in the structure and growth of animals and plants. Sydenham, London

van Leeuwenhoek A (1678) Microscopical observations of the structure of teeth and other bones. Philos Trans R Soc Lond 12:1002–1003

Vesalius A (1543) De humani corporis fabrica. Johannes Oporinus, Basel

Vesalius A (1551) Anatomia: Ein kurtzer Auszug der beschreibung, aller glider menschlichs Leybs aus den buchern des Hochgelerten Hern D. Andree Vesalij von Brüssel Nürnberg: Jul. Paulo Fabricio

Virchow R (1850) Knochen- und Knorpelkörperchen. Verh Physik med Ges Würzburg 1:193–197

von Meyer H (1867) Die Architektur der Spongiosa. Arch Anat Physiol 34:615–628

Weber W, Weber E (1836) Mechanik der menschlichen Gehwerkzeuge. In: Merkel F, Fischer O (1894) Wilhelm Weber's Werk; Kgl Ges d Wiss Göttingen (ed). Springer, Berlin

Weidenreich F (1930) Das Knochengewebe. In: Moellendorff W von (Hrg): Handbuch der mikroskopischen Anatomie des Menschen; II: Die Gewebe; 2. Teil: Stützgewebe-Knochengewebe-Skeletsystem. Julius Springer, Berlin

Wolff J (1892) Das Gesetz der Transformation der Knochen. Hirschwald, Berlin

Microscopical Anatomy

2.1 Hyaline Cartilage

The hyaline articular cartilage appears remarkably smooth, both macroscopically and on examination by light microscopy (LM) or transmission electron microscopy (TEM), and even – after introduction of the cold stage – in the scanning electron microscope (Hunter 1743; Davies et al. 1962; Ghadially and Roy 1969; Draenert and Draenert 1979; Draenert et al. 2002). Hyaline cartilage is firmly anchored in the bony baseplate which is best demonstrated in histological studies with sections which have been processed under load (Fig. 2.1). Undulations, pits, and humps as surface characteristics are considered artifacts by drying (Clarke 1971a, b, c; Ghadially et al. 1976.1977; Draenert and Draenert 1979; Draenert et al. 2002).

A tissue such as hyaline cartilage, which contains up to 70% water and which is known to easily lose proteoglycans during processing (Cameron et al. 1976), is best investigated in the frozen, non-dehydrated state (Draenert et al. 2002; Fig. 2.2). The water content of cartilage ranges from 65% to over 80% in the upper layers facing the joint (Venn and Maroudas 1977). Rosenberg et al. (1970, 1975) developed macromolecular models of protein polysaccharides. Articular cartilage may be considered as a visco- or poro-elastic fiber-composite material (Becerra et al. 2010). Recent studies on the friction coefficient of articular cartilage showed that the main boundary lubricant is the SZP molecule, the Superficial Zone Protein (Chan et al. 2010).

The scanning electron microscope probably best shows the three-dimensional structure of the tissue. A layer of ground substance free of fibers

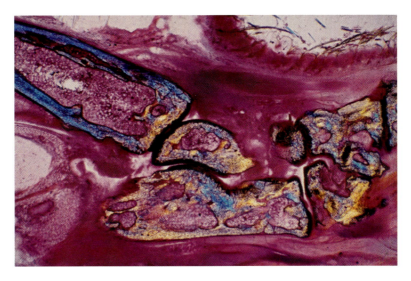

Fig. 2.1 Longitudinal section of a mouse's ankle and foot under load: the cartilage is firmly anchored with its fibers onto the bony baseplate

Fig. 2.2 Cold stage, developed in the ZOW Munich in order to study cartilage in a "nondehydrated" stage (DFG support)

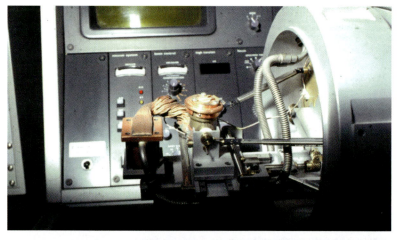

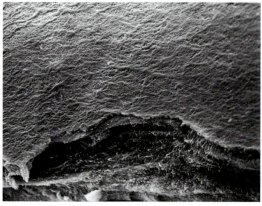

Fig. 2.3 View of the hyaline cartilage: It is smooth, without undulations, pits, and humps, revealing a lamina splendens. SEM of a freeze-dried, freeze-fractured femoral head of a rat in the PSEM 500, 25 kV, 200 Å Au. Horizontal field width = 40 μm

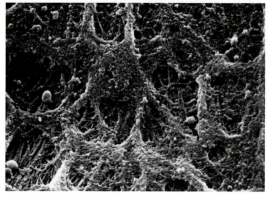

Fig. 2.4 Partially freed-fiber pattern of the tangential fiber layer of a rat's femoral head. Ice crystal processing: there is a well-organized, tangentially oriented fiber pattern visible. SEM of a freeze-dried specimen in the PSEM 500, 25 kV, 200 Å. Horizontal field width = 12 μm

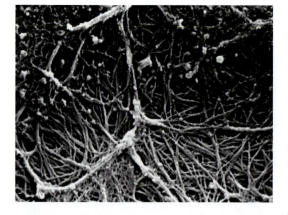

Fig. 2.5 Exposed fibers of the tangential layer of hyaline cartilage of a rat's femoral head. Ice crystal processing: there is a well-organized, tangentially oriented fiber pattern visible. A canal system is revealed through the fiber pattern. SEM of a freeze-dried specimen in the PSEM 500, 25 kV, 200 Å. Horizontal field width = 12 μm

covers the surface (*lamina splendens*) (Fig. 2.3). In the electron microscope, it is revealed that the ground substance is grouted over a tangential network of collagenous fibers (Figs. 2.4 and 2.5).

The tangential layer of fibers was arched like a dome over the underlying structures. Under this dome, cell columns arched revealing disklike cells adjacent to the tangential fiber layer. Specimen processed at the cold stage showed no shrinkage at all (Fig. 2.6). In the arch, oval cells appear followed by isogenous cell groups (Figs. 2.7 and 2.8).

The surface of the cartilage baseplate is tremendously enlarged and best presented in the scanning electron microscope (Fig. 2.9).

2.2 Epiphyseal Cancellous Bone

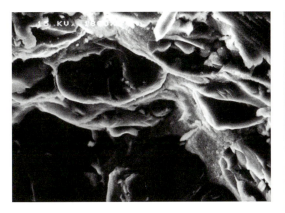

Fig. 2.6 Tangential cell layer in a nondehydrated stage: There is no shrinkage at all. The chondrocytes fill the fiber basket completely and act as hydraulic elements. SEM of a frozen nondehydrated specimen in the PSEM 500, equipped with a cold stage, 25 kV, 200 Å. Horizontal field width = 35 μm

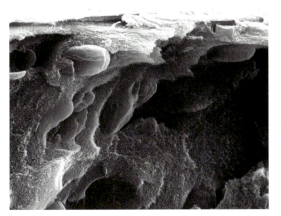

Fig. 2.7 Cell arch in a freeze-dried and freeze-fractured sample of a rat's femoral head in the SEM. The cell membrane is slightly folded due to the drying process. SEM of a freeze-dried specimen in the PSEM 500, 25 kV, 200 Å. Horizontal field width = 60 μm

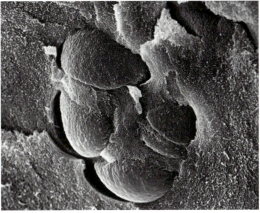

Fig. 2.8 Isogenous cell group of the deeper layer in a freeze-dried and freeze-fractured sample of a rat's femoral head in the SEM. Between cell membrane and fiber basket, a slight gap has developed due to the drying process. SEM of a freeze-dried specimen in the PSEM 500, 25 kV, 200 Å. Horizontal field width = 35 μm

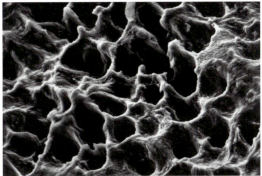

Fig. 2.9 View of the bony cartilage baseplate: A huge surface enlargement with deep pits is revealed. SEM of an air-dried specimen of a rat's femoral head corroded with Na_2O_2 and documented in the PSEM 500, 25 kV, 200 Å. Horizontal field width = 80 μm

2.2 Epiphyseal Cancellous Bone

The tissue of the epiphyses consists of hyaline cartilage connected with the perichondrium to the diaphyseal tube, forming in between the growth plate and toward the perichondrium the "encoche d'ossification" Ranvier (1873). Genetically determined, a vascularized connective tissue grows in from the perichondrium and forms the ossification center in the middle of the epiphysis (Schenk 1978). The enchondral ossification grows radially, forming the load-bearing epiphyseal joint component.

The epiphysis is comprised of the compact cartilage baseplate – cementing all fiber bundles of the hyaline cartilage – and the cancellous bone with strong arches of bone forming a vault (Fig. 2.10). Depending on the load acting on it, the cartilage baseplate can be thin, containing thin arches of cancellous bone, i.e., in the epiphyseal part of the phalanges (Fig. 2.11), or very compact, as revealed in the femoral head (Fig. 2.12). In all cases, the strength of the lamellae depends upon the load acting on it; based on Wolff's Law (1892), an interpretation of the architecture of the cancellous bone, i.e., through

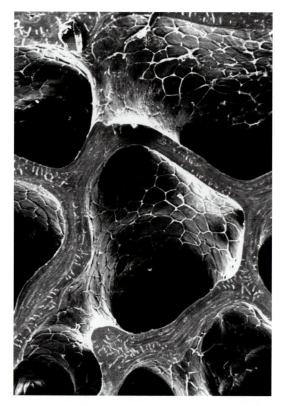

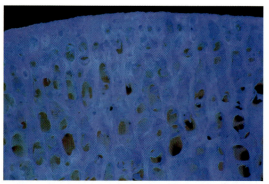

Fig. 2.12 Frontal section through a corroded femoral head of a 50-year-old man: the compact cartilage baseplate of a human femoral head is presented, supported by strong trabeculae comprising bone marrow spaces of distally increasing diameter. Ground section in incident fluorescent light. Horizontal field width = 650 µm

Fig. 2.10 Epiphyseal cancellous bone of a dog's tibial head: the shell-like structure of the cancellous bone is apparent. MMA-deplastified sample in the SEM. SEM of an air-dried specimen of a deplastified longitudinal ground section cleaned with pressurized air and documented in the PSEM 500, 50 kV, 200 Å. Horizontal field width = 650 µm

the center of rotation of the femoral head, can be made (Fig. 2.13). The arterial vascularization of the epiphyses shows a lot of variables and is not yet comprehensively studied and documented. The arterial blood supply of the epiphysis plays a major role in all osteonecroses and is of utmost importance for the surgical approach for fracture treatment, i.e., the anterolateral approach for fractures of the lateral tibial condyle. The anatomy in that special topographical compartment was recently worked out (Hannouche et al. 2006). The deep branch of the medial femoral circumflex artery is considered of similar importance to

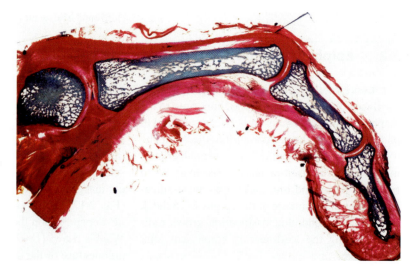

Fig. 2.11 Longitudinal section of a limb chain with joints, revealing the concave and convex delicate baseplate of the cartilage. Ground section of a human index finger, nondemineralized MMA-embedded ground section, basic fuchsine staining. Horizontal field width = 10 cm

2.3 Metaphyseal Cancellous Bone

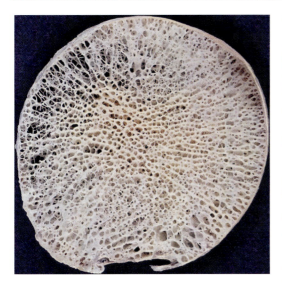

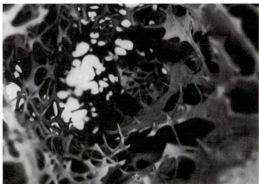

Fig. 2.13 Cross section through the center of rotation of a human femoral head: the orientation of the trabeculae resembles the balance wheel of a clock resisting strain acting upon it in a sagittal direction during walking. Two-millimeter-thick corroded cross section under the microscope. Horizontal field width = 55 mm. Leitz: Aristophot

Fig. 2.14 View of the shell-like cancellous bone of the proximal metaphysis of a human femur: The medullary cavity is revealed with its wall-like shells. Corroded proximal femur of a 50-year-old man with resected femoral head and resected distal tube. Cleaned marrow spaces. Documentation was performed under the microscope using incident and transmitted light. Leitz: Macrozoom. Horizontal field width = 90 mm

avoid or to understand the development of femoral head necrosis, i.e., for the surgical dislocation of the hip (Gautier et al. 2000; Ganz et al. 2001).

2.3 Metaphyseal Cancellous Bone

The shell-like structure of all bone subunits guarantees the largest possible surface area for resorption and, in the same way, its reinforcement. Toward the metaphysis, the shell-like walls of the cancellous bone become thinner and tubelike and well pronounced near the cortex of the proximal femur (Fig. 2.14) and along the metaphyseal cortical wall (Fig. 2.15). The thickness of a metaphyseal cancellous bone trabecula ranges between 80 and 100 μm, whereas the epiphyseal one is stronger and on average 250 μm thick. Sharpey's fiber bundles take a divergent spiral course inside the bone (Weidenreich 1922). The joint capsule, their reinforcements, ligaments, and tendons follow this principle, mainly in the metaphyseal compartment. A ligament or tendon substitute pulled through a drilled channel of a bone will

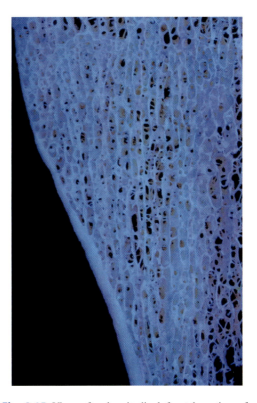

Fig. 2.15 View of a longitudinal frontal section of a human lateral femoral metaphysis. The shell-like cancellous bone comprises marrow spaces with a distally increasing diameter (1,000 μm). Corroded and cleaned sample from the lateral femoral metaphysis of a 50-year-old man, 2 mm thick, documented in incident fluorescent light. Horizontal field width = 15 mm. Leitz: Makrozoom

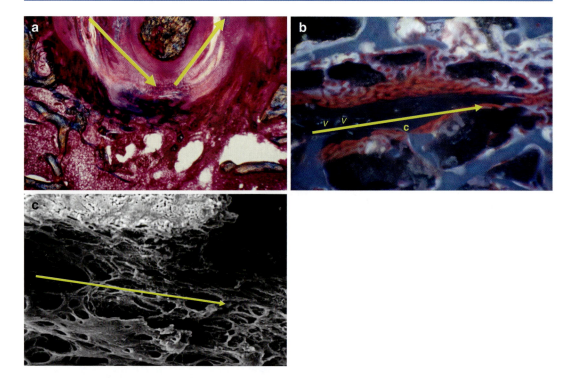

Fig. 2.16 (**a**) Cross section of a V-shaped drill hole anchorage of a ligament plastic: the cutis is pulled through a V-shaped drill hole (*arrows*); 6 weeks after the operation on a rabbit's tibial head, there is nearly no pronounced bony anchorage. MMA-embedded cross section in polarized transmitted light; alkaline fuchsine staining. Horizontal field width = 12 mm. Leitz: Orthoplan; Apochromat 2.5×. (**b**) Cross section of a sandwich anchorage of a cutis plastic in a rabbit's tibial head: the sandwich gap was performed with a 300-μm saw blade by hand. The sandwich was closed by a miniscrew which pinched the cutis between bone surfaces (*arrow*). Three weeks after the operation, the cutis (*c*) is well vascularized and bony integrated from both sides. The vessels show a light blue fluorescence (*v*); the bony anchorage took place in the second and third week (*blue* and *red label*); in the first week (*yellow label*), the recipient bed was reinforced. MMA-embedded cross section in incident fluorescent light; basic fuchsine staining. UV-filter. Horizontal field width = 1,500 μm; Leitz: Orthoplan; Apochromat 4×. (**c**) Corroded cross section of (**c**) in the SEM: the newly formed bone is oriented along the path of fibers of the cutis (*arrow*), which has been removed by corrosion. The strong bony anchorage is well pronounced. Na_2O_2 processing, cleaning with gentle jet of a jet lavage; air-dried specimen. 200 Å gold sputtering. PSEM 500, 50 kV. Horizontal field width = 150 μm

not be bony anchored by newly formed bone because the fibers converge, concentrating stress instead of distributing it (Draenert et al. 1981). The principle of a divergent course should be considered for the replantation operation, for which there are principally two possibilities: the sandwich technique, (Fig. 2.16a–c; Draenert et al. 1981) or the bone dowelling technique, i.e., the bone–tendon–bone procedure replacing the ACL in the knee joint (Fig. 2.17a–e).

2.3 Metaphyseal Cancellous Bone

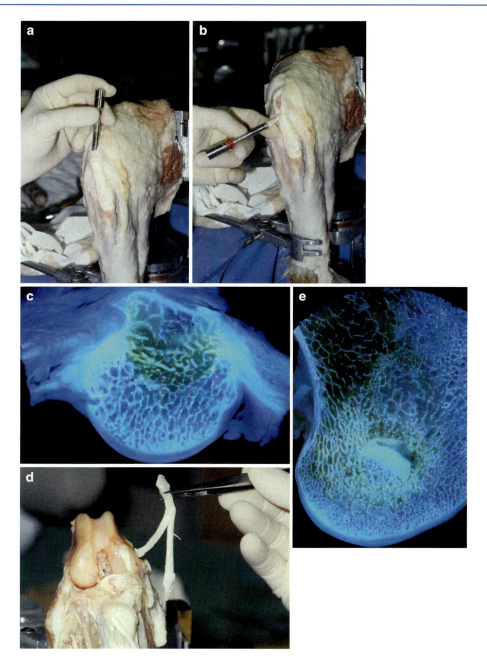

Fig. 2.17 (**a**, **b**) Animal experiment (Gerber, London) in a shepherd dog with the SDI procedure: a very precise wet-grinding process gathers the bone-tendon-bone graft. Preoperative planning in a dog's cadaver bone, just before the patellar tendon is cut. Leica: Kodak prof. 64. (**c**) Cross section through the dog's patella: a press-fit graft, gathered from the iliac crest and bony healed after 4 weeks, refills the donor bed. Fresh cross section in incident fluorescent light reveals the *yellow label* of the first and second postoperative week. Horizontal field width = 22.5 mm. ZOW: *HIIFL* high intensity incident fluorescent light. (**d**) Double bundle plastic using the outside-in technique in a preoperative dog's cadaver planning: the patellar tendon, as well as the bony shell of the tuberositas patellae, is split; both bundles are anchored in the tibial head and twisted 30–45°. (**e**) Bony integration of the patellar bone plug revealing the sandwich incorporation of the fiber layer in the ground canal of the lateral femoral condyle. Insertion was performed in a press-fit manner using the SDI technique. A fresh sagittal section in incident fluorescent light reveals the *yellow label* of the first and second postoperative week. Horizontal field width = 19 mm. ZOW: *HIIFL* high intensity incident fluorescent light

References

Becerra J, Andrades JA, Guerado E et al (2010) Articular cartilage: structure and regeneration. Tissue Eng 16:617–627

Cameron CHS, Gardner DL, Longmore RB (1976) The preparation of human articular cartilage for SEM. J Microsc 108:1–12

Chan SM, Neu CP, Duraine G et al (2010) Atomic force microscope investigation of the boundary-lubricant layer in articular cartilage. Osteoarthritis Cartilage 18:956–963

Clarke IC (1971a) Human articular surface contours and related surface depression. Frequency studies. Ann Rheum Dis 30:15–23

Clarke IC (1971b) A method for the replication of the articular cartilage surfaces suitable for the scanning electron microscope. J Microsc 93:67–71

Clarke IC (1971c) Surface characteristics of human articular cartilage. A SEM study. J Anat 108:23–30

Davies VD, Barnett CH, Cochrane W et al (1962) Electron microscopy of articular cartilage in the young adult rabbit. Ann Rheum Dis 21:11–22

Draenert Y, Draenert K (1979) Freeze-drying of articular cartilage. Scanning 2:57–71

Draenert K, Draenert Y, Springorum HW et al (1981) Histo-Morphologie des Spongiosadefektes und die Heilung des autologen Spongiosatransplantates. In: Cotta H, Martini AK (eds) Implantate und Transplantate in der Plastischen und Wiederherstellungschirurgie. Springer, Berlin

Draenert K, Draenert Y, Bombelli R et al (2002) La guarigione primaria della cartilagine e dell'osso spugnoso ed il suo significato clinico. In: Pipino F (ed) G I O T 28:531–539

Ganz R, Gill TJ, Gautier E et al (2001) Surgical dislocation of the adult hip. A technique with full access to the femoral head and acetabulum without the risk of avascular necrosis. J Bone Joint Surg 83-B:1119–1124

Gautier E, Ganz K, Krügel N et al (2000) Anatomy of the medial femoral circumflex artery and its surgical implications. J Bone Joint Surg 82-B:679–683

Ghadially FN, Roy S (1969) Ultrastructure of synovial joints in health and diseases. Livingstone, London, pp 40–86

Ghadially FN, Ghadially JA, Oryschak AF et al (1976) Experimental production of ridges on rabbit articular cartilage. J Anat 121:119–132

Ghadially FN, Thomas I, Oryschak AF et al (1977) Long-term results of superficial defects in articular cartilage. J Pathol 121:213–222

Hannouche D, Duparc F, Beaufils P (2006) The arterial vascularization of the lateral tibial condyle: anatomy and surgical application. Surg Radiol Anat 28:38–45

Hunter W (1743) Of the structures and diseases of articulating cartilage. Philos Trans R Soc Lond (Biol) 42:514–521

Ranvier L (1873) Quelque faits relatifs au dévelopment du tissus osseux. Comptes rendus Acad Sci 77:1105–1109

Rosenberg L, Hellmann W, Kleinschmidt AK (1970) Macromolecular models of protein polysaccharides from bovine nasal cartilage based on electron microscopic studies. J Biol Chem 245:4123–4130

Rosenberg L, Hellmann W, Kleinschmidt AK (1975) Electron microscopic studies of proteoglycan aggregates from bovine articular cartilage. J Biol Chem 250:1877–1883

Schenk R (1978) Histomorphologische und physiologische Grundlagen des Skelettwachstums. In: Weber BG, Brunner Ch, Freuler F (eds) Die Frakturbehandlung bei Kindern und Jugendlichen. Springer, Berlin

Venn M, Maroudas A (1977) Chemical composition and swelling of normal and osteoarthritic femoral head cartilage. I. Chemical comp. Ann Rheum Dis 36:121–129

Weidenreich F (1922) Über die Beziehungen zwischen Muskelapparat und Knochen und dem Charakter des Knochengewebes. Erg H Anat Anz 55:28–53

Wolff J (1892) Das Gesetz der Transformation der Knochen. Hirschwald, Berlin

Bone Growth

3.1 Epiphyseal Growth

The development of the ossification center in the epiphyseal ends of long bones may be genetically determined (Schenk 1978); it exists, however, in close relationship to the biomechanical stress acting upon it. The process of vascularization has been well studied and was first described by Maximow (1910), who found that embryogenic tissue of the inner perichondrium, rich in vascularization, grows into the cartilage and forms after resorption of the cartilage by chondroclasts (Dantschakoff 1909), the primary medullary cavity according to Hammar (1901). The osteoprogenitor cells of the primary bone marrow derive from the perivascular ingrowing embryogenic tissue. The transition from the epiphysis to the diaphyseal tube is made by the "rainure circulaire" or "encoche d'ossification" of Ranvier (1873), responsible for the transversal growth of the growth plate in between the epiphysis and the diaphysis. The first scaffold is woven of felt bone replacing the cartilage. Under load, lamellar reinforcement and remodeling take place and form a radially growing epiphyseal spongiosa, revealing a bony cartilage baseplate toward the joint supporting the hyaline joint cartilage, as well as a baseplate toward the growth plate (Fig. 3.1). The anchoring plate of the epiphysis toward the growth plate reveals an enormous surface enlargement (Fig. 3.2) on the bottom of which a network of a venous drainage system is presented (Fig. 3.3) (Draenert and Draenert 1985). The growth plate itself is part of the metaphysis. The corrosion casts of the vasculature present a widely branching, regular vascular network which rests on the entire plate and is protected by the bony anchoring protuberances. These vessels are wide, thin-walled venous capillaries with varying morphology which correspond to the sinusoids of the bone marrow, presenting a course at a constant distance to the bone surface. The epiphyseal growth takes place by bone apposition and resorption, an osseous shift, and drift (Enlow 1963). Compared to the epiphysis, the apophysis is comprised of the same components (Fig. 3.4). The architecture of the cancellous bone, however, looks different, and instead of the hyaline cartilage of the joint, Sharpey's fibers of the inserting

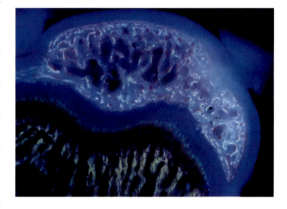

Fig. 3.1 Bony shift and apposition in a growing rabbit's femoral epiphysis: the four-colored labels indicate the shift of the epiphyseal shape during 4-week growth. The same label appears as a band label along the growth plate. Fresh frontal section is documented in the HIIFL microscope (UV-light). Horizontal field width = 8 mm

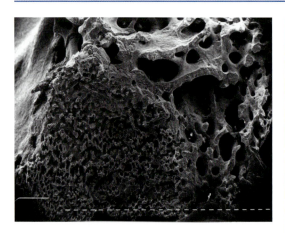

Fig. 3.2 View of the bony baseplate of the epiphysis which reveals the anchoring bone stock of the compact baseplate. A specimen in the SEM, which is comprised of bone together with the replica of the vasculature. The vasculature was injected with a MMA resin (Mercox®, Vilene Cy., Japan), and the specimen was corroded, carefully cleaned, and sputtered with gold (200 Å). PSEM 500, 50 kV. Horizontal field width = 6 mm

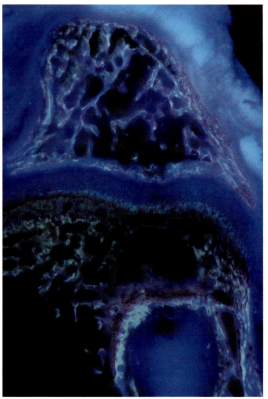

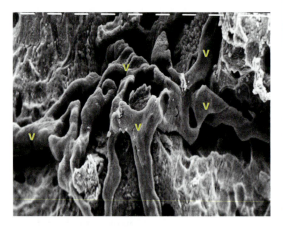

Fig. 3.3 View of the epiphyseal anchoring plate revealing a complete venous network of vessels (*v*) at a constant distance to the bone, measuring 20 µm. Bone-vasculature specimen in the SEM. The vasculature was injected with a MMA resin (Mercox®, Vilene Cy., Japan), and the specimen was corroded, carefully cleaned, and sputtered with gold (200 Å). PSEM 500, 50 kV. Horizontal field width = 200 µm

Fig. 3.4 Bony shift and apposition in a growing rabbit's femoral apophysis: The four-colored labels indicate the shift of the apophyseal shape during 4-week growth. The architecture of the internal structure is obviously different compared with the epiphysis. The morphology of the anchoring in the growth plate reveals no difference. The same label appears as a band label along the growth plate. Fresh frontal section in the HIIFL microscope (UV-light). Horizontal field width = 8 mm

musculature form the baseplate on the other end. Tension forces acting on the apophysis construct its scaffold.

3.2 Metaphyseal Growth

The growth of the metaphysis is presented like an open V-shape, bearing the growth plate and inserted into the tube of the diaphysis (Fig. 3.5). Bone apposition always starts inside the medullary cavity and crosses all bone structures in a centrifugal direction, finally forming the next plateau of the growth plate (Fig. 3.5). The construction can form a symmetrical V-shape, as seen in the knee (Fig. 3.6), or an asymmetrical,

3.2 Metaphyseal Growth

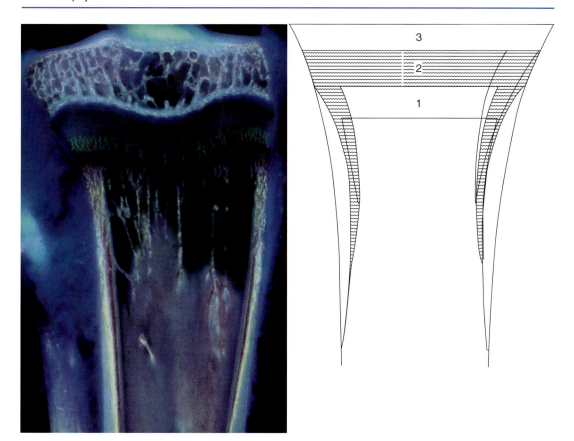

Fig. 3.5 The V-shapes of the proximal tibial metaphyses are put together in such a way that the formation of new bone starts along the inner wall of the medullary cavity, crosses the entire thickness of the metaphyseal cortex, and forms the new growth plate, resembling an overhanging balcony. The label can be followed starting with the *1 yellow*, *2 red*, and *3 green label*, continuously applied during 4 weeks. A fresh frontal section through a growing rabbit's tibial bone was documented in the HIIFL microscope in UV-light (ZOW)

eccentric shape, like the formation of the femoral neck in the proximal femur (Fig. 3.7a). The epiphyses exceed the metaphyses and biomechanically influence the "encoche" and the metaphyseal and diaphyseal bone formation.

The wall of the metaphyseal V-shape corresponds in its proximal segment spongious in form (Fig. 3.7b) and in its distal part to longitudinal tubes (Fig. 3.7c). The new bone formation of the femoral neck follows a course that begins along the medullary canal, interweaves thoroughly the spongious structure, and forms the outer layer of the neck, converting part of the spongious structure to compact bone (Fig. 3.8a, b).

McLean and Bloom (1940) divided the growth plate into four microscopic anatomic zones, a classification which is still used: (1 = toward the joint) the zone of resting cartilage, (2) the zone of proliferation, (3) the zone of mature or even hypertrophic cartilage, (4) and the zone of mineralized cartilage. The cells of the first two layers are capable of proliferation (Kember 1960). The nutrient vessels of the growth plate derive from the nutrient main arteries of the tibia and the metaphyseal arteries. Rami with a horizontal course branched off from the stronger arterial vessels at the level of the primary spongiosa trabeculae. These rami ascended with a regular and

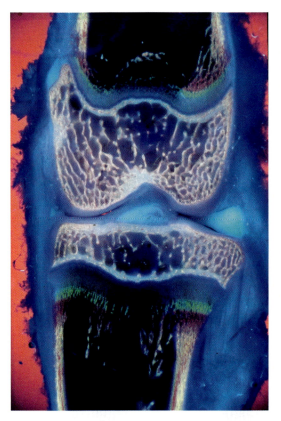

Fig. 3.6 View of a growing joint of a rabbit, continuously labeled over 4 weeks. The growth pattern of the epiphyses is clearly differentiated against the metaphyseal one. The growth of the epiphyses is marked by apposition and shift, whereas the metaphyseal growth is designed by newly formed and overlapping V-shapes. Fresh, frontal section through a growing rabbit's knee joint. Documentation was performed in the HIIFL microscope in UV-light (ZOW)

vertical course into the intertrabecular medullary spaces beneath the plate's cartilage with arterial capillaries branching off at nearly right angles (Fig. 3.9). The arterial vessels with a horizontal course were connected to the metaphyseal centripetal arterial influxes; they were found at the level of the vertical spongiosa trabeculae of the metaphysis. These trabeculae ended in the free medullary cavity. The arterial capillaries – without branching off further – could be followed into the cartilage's zone of mineralization. The terminal capillaries formed various sprouts, which forged ahead toward the cartilage (Fig. 3.10). These end capillaries were opposed to a clearly defined venous drainage system.

3.3 Diaphyseal Growth

The ossification of the tube of long bones begins with a periosteal newly formed bone sleeve. The bone sleeve extends toward both ends in a funnel-shaped manner, in which the metaphyseal V-shape formations are taken up. The appositional periosteal growth is combined with an "endosteal" resorption by osteoclasts (Fig. 3.11a, b). The cross section is directly correlated to the biomechanical impact by the load axis, which shifts during growth. As a result, the bony tube is constantly changing its matter through remodeling processes. The basic underlying principle is well described as osseous drift (Enlow 1963).

3.3 Diaphyseal Growth

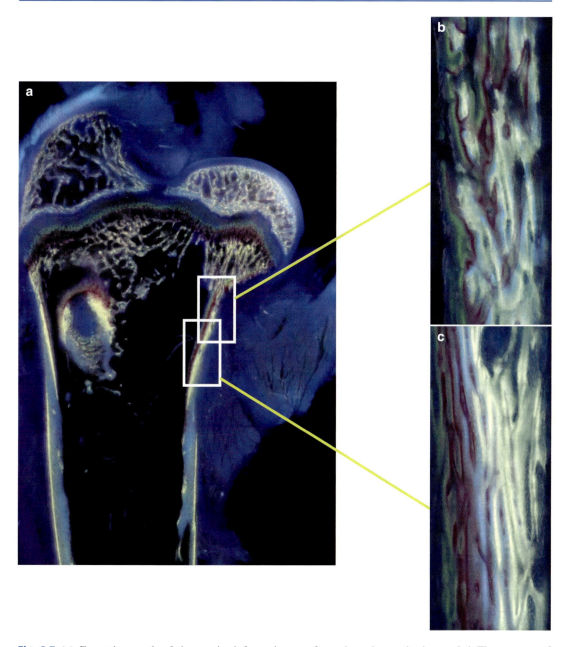

Fig. 3.7 (**a**) Eccentric growth of the proximal femoral metaphysis reveals the more spongious lamellar reinforcement in its proximal part (**b**) and the concentrated lamellar arrangement along the tube of the femur (**c**). The four labels, one for each week, are clearly revealed. The sequence of labeling was *yellow*, *blue*, *red*, and finally *green*. A fresh, frontal section through a growing rabbit's femoral bone was documented in the HIIFL microscope in UV-light (ZOW)

Fig. 3.8 (**a**, **b**) View of the formation of the femoral neck. The growth plate always eccentrically overlaps the underlying cortical tube. The formation of the new bone always starts inside the medullary canal, crosses through the cortex, and forms the balcony of the femoral neck, which carries the epiphysis of the femoral head. A fresh frontal section through a growing rabbit's tibial bone was documented in the HIIFL microscope in UV-light (ZOW) *1 yellow, 2 red, 3 green*

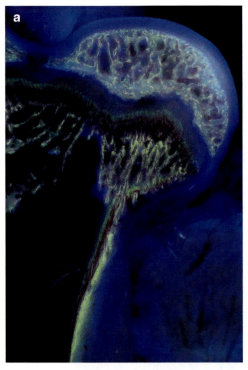
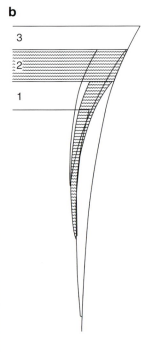

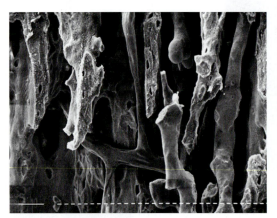

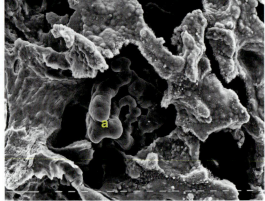

Fig. 3.9 Arterial blood supply of the growth plate: an arteriole branches off in arterial capillaries going straight upward to the growth plate. A specimen in the SEM comprised of bone together with the replica of the vasculature. The vascular network was injected with a MMA resin (Mercox®, Vilene Cy., Japan) and the specimen corroded, carefully cleaned, and sputtered with gold (200 Å). PSEM 500, 50 kV. Horizontal field width = 800 μm

Fig. 3.10 View of the growth plate of the bone-vasculature specimen revealing the end pieces of the arterial capillaries (*a*). The cartilage has been removed. A specimen in the SEM comprised of bone together with the replica of the vasculature. The vascular network was injected with a MMA resin (Mercox®, Vilene Cy., Japan) and the specimen corroded, carefully cleaned, and sputtered with gold (200 Å). PSEM 500, 50 kV. Horizontal field width = 400 μm

Fig. 3.11 (**a**, **b**) The labeling of the diaphyseal tube looks different compared with the metaphysis. The V-shape is still distinctly visible along the inner wall of the medullary cavity. In addition to that formation, the periosteal apposition is pronounced (**b**). *1 yellow label*, *2 blue label*, *3 red label*. Fresh frontal section through a growing rabbit's tibial bone, documented in the HIIFL microscope in UV-light (ZOW)

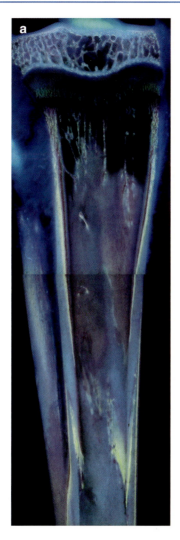
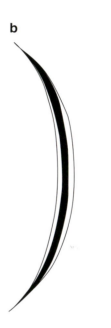
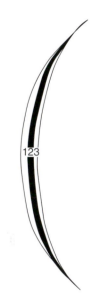

References

Dantschakoff W (1909) Über die Entwicklung des Knochenmarks bei den Vögeln und über dessen Veränderungen bei Blutentziehungen und Ernährungsstörungen. Arch mikr Anat 74:855–926

Draenert K, Draenert Y (1985) The role of the vessels in the growth plate: morphological examination. Scanning electron microscopy, vol I. SEM Inc, Chicago, pp 339–344

Enlow DH (1963) Principles of bone remodeling. Thomas, Springfield

Hammar J (1901) Primäres und rotes Knochenmark. Anat Anz 19:567–570

Kember NF (1960) Cell division in endochondral ossification. A study of cell proliferation in rat bones by the method of tritiated thymidine autoradiography. J Bone Joint Surg 42-B:824–839

Maximow A (1910) Untersuchungen über Blut und Bindegewebe. III. Die embryonale Histogenese des Knochenmarks der Säugetiere. Arch mikr Anat 76:1–113

McLean FC, Blom W (1940) Calcification and ossification. Calcification in the normal growing bone. Anat Rec 78:333–359

Ranvier L (1873) Quelque faits relatifs au dévelopment du tissus osseux. Comptes rendus Acad Sci 77: 1105–1109

Schenk R (1978) Histomorphologische und physiologische Grundlagen des Skelettwachstums. In: Weber BG, Brunner CH, Freuler F (eds) Die Frakturbehandlung bei Kindern und Jugendlichen. Springer, Berlin

Regeneration and Healing

4.1 Hyaline Cartilage

There are two models for studying degradation and lamination of hyaline articular cartilage: the Silberberg mouse (Silberberg et al. 1965a, b) and the ACL-cut model on animals (Draenert and Draenert 1981). The Silberberg mouse develops during the first year of severe varus osteoarthritis in the knee joint. The varus deformation is induced by hormones. The osteoarthritis reveals all signs of a progredient degradation of the joint with the development of osteophytes (Fig. 4.1) and destruction of the hyaline cartilage, which is abraded in layers (Figs. 4.2 and 4.3). Simultaneous with the destruction, reparation processes with newly produced ground substance and proliferating cells can be observed (Fig. 4.4).

The experimental model on rats, in which the ACL was cut, revealed a whirl-like ulceration with rupture of the tangential fiber layer (Fig. 4.5) in the center of the medial condyle and less pronounced on the kissing tibial head after 6 months. The repair processes of articular cartilage depend on the depth of the lesion. Up to 1 mm a restitutio ad integrum was observed in animal experiments, whereas 2-mm-deep defects showed a significant lower score (Sun et al. 2011). There is an intrinsic tissue repair of the articular surfaces, which can be influenced on a molecular basis, i.e., with BMP 7 or BMP 2 and TGF-ß (Frenkel et al. 2000; Dell'accio and Vincent 2010; Tokuhara et al.

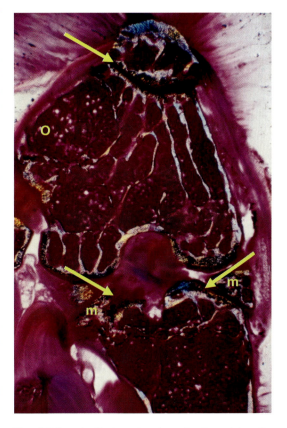

Fig. 4.1 Longitudinal section through a knee joint of a Silberberg mouse suffering severe osteoarthritis comprising destruction of the tibial plateau, osteophytes (*O*), ossification of the menisci (*m*), and loss of cartilage (*arrows*). One year of age. MMA-embedded cross section stained with basic fuchsine and documented in the polarized path of rays in the Orthoplan (Leitz). Horizontal field width = 6 mm

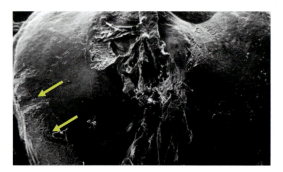

Fig. 4.2 View of the tibial plateau of a Silberberg mouse, 1 year of age: the hyaline cartilage appears rough and irregular and more pronounced along the edges of the plateau (*arrows*). Tangential fiber layer in a freeze-dried stage: There is no shrinkage. SEM of a freeze-dried specimen in the PSEM 500, 25 kV, 200 Å Au. Horizontal field width = 3 mm

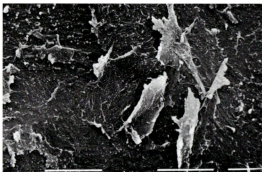

Fig. 4.4 View of the more centralized surface of the hyaline cartilage of the lateral tibial plateau. Reparation processes are visible with new formation of ground substance and collagen fibers forming a tangential layer. SEM of a freeze-dried specimen in the PSEM 500, 25 kV, 200 Å Au. Horizontal field width = 50 μm

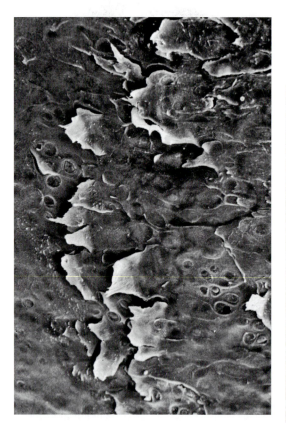

Fig. 4.3 Degradation in layers of the hyaline cartilage in a 1-year-old Silberberg mouse: the chondrocytes have been sheared away; their baskets are empty (*arrows*). The lateral condyle of the tibial plateau is presented. At that stage, the mouse shows severe varus deformity. SEM of a freeze-dried specimen in the PSEM 500, 25 kV, 200 Å Au. Horizontal field width = 360 μm

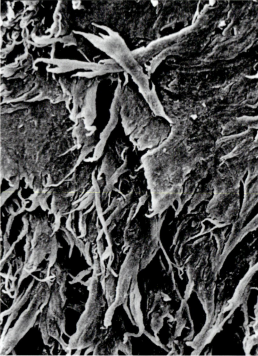

Fig. 4.5 View of a medial tibial plateau of a rat in which the ACL had been cut 4 weeks prior: the tangential fiber layer is ruptured in the center of the medial tibial plateau. SEM of a freeze-dried specimen in the PSEM 500, 25 kV, 200 Å Au. Horizontal field width = 60 μm

2010; Draenert et al. 2012). It could be shown on the one side that tissue-specific stem cells, responding to molecular signals (Karlsson and Lindahl 2009), participate in repair processes following injury and, on the other side, that those adult tissues loose that potential in part, showing only a low regeneration capacity compared with fetal, tissue-specific stem cells (Quintin et al. 2010; Otsuki et al. 2010).

Table 4.1 Topography of osteo-cartilage fractures

Acetabulum	Ragnarsson et al. (1992)
Hip	Tehranzadeh et al. (1990)
Metatarsal and phalanges	Jones (1987); Dutkowsky and Freeman (1989)
Hallux	Wertheimer and Balzsy (1992)
Shoulder	Blasier and Burkus (1988); Zilch and Talke (1987)
Hand	Green and O'Brien (1980); Bohart et al. (1982); Stripling (1982); McElfresh and Dobyns (1983); Saffar (1984); Larson et al. (1987); Light and Ogden (1988)

4.2 Epiphyseal Bone

The epiphyseal fracture in most cases concerns osteocartilaginous fragments which are diagnosed by arthroscopy due to the hemarthrosis (Schild and Ahlers 1987; Butler and Andrews 1988; Stanitski et al. 1993; Feder and Schonholtz 1992; Barber and Prudich 1993). Especially in the ankle, the arthroscopy detected many osteochondral fractures (Parisien and Vangsness 1985). The ankle joint is often traumatized in high-level athletes (Hontas et al. 1986). The osteochondral fractures of the talus dome are of central importance (Huylebroek et al. 1985). The relationship between trauma and the osteochondritis dissecans is discussed (Mazel et al. 1986). The classification of Berndt and Harty (1959) is still applied. There is a high level of posttraumatic osteoarthritis reported (Pettine and Morrey 1987). The inverted osteochondral fracture is diagnosed by means of a CT scan and has to be operated on immediately (Kenny 1981; Holzheimer und Kunze 1987). In the knee joint, luxation of the patella is frequently accompanied by osteochondral fracture (Runow 1983), even of the patella itself (Miligram 1985; Keller et al. 1985). The main reasons for osteochondral fractures combined with the dislocation of the patella are high-energy traumata (Maquire and Canale 1993; Gilbert et al. 1993). Osteochondral fractures also comprise the avulsion fracture of the cruciate ligaments (Noyes et al. 1980). Both have to be operated on within a short time (Bachelin and Bugmann 1988; Wasilewski and Frankl 1992).

The femoral condyles – in children the medial one, in adults more often the lateral condyle – are often diagnosed in athletes and following car accidents (Torg et al. 1981; Gilley et al. 1981; Wilson and Scranton 1990). Nearly all structures of the glenoid joint can be involved (Butler and Andrews 1988; Mink and Deutsch 1989; Wilson and Scranton 1990; Hardaker et al. 1990; Lewis and Foster 1990; Bomberg and McGinty 1990; Vellet et al. 1991; Paar and Boszotta 1991; Isaacs and Schreiber 1992; Barber and Prudich 1993; Stanitski et al. 1993; Laredo et al. 1993). In car accidents, 25% of the fractures are chondral and 75% are osteochondral fractures (Paar and Boszotta 1991).

Chondral and osteochondral fractures can occur in all glenoid joints and are more often diagnosed today due to the arthroscopy, the CT scan, or NMR (Table 4.1).

Small osteochondral fragments are often excised (Ove et al. 1989; Frank et al. 1989; Bohart et al. 1982; Hämmerle and Jacob 1980). Apart from that, the treatments were very varied (Table 4.2).

Osteocartilage fragments which are at least 8 mm thick are best fixated with one or two autologous osteocartilage dowels (Fig. 4.6). The dowelling method is considered superior compared with screw fixation (Fig. 4.7) because a second intervention can be avoided, and in addition, screws traumatize the hyaline cartilage on both sides. The fracture healed after 4 weeks and, after 3 months, even the hyaline cartilage had healed primarily in a contact healing of bone and cartilage (Fig. 4.8).

In joint reconstructions with autologous or related fresh homologous cartilage-bone grafts, the primary contact healing could be shown as well after 4 weeks (Figs. 4.9, 4.10, and 4.11). The histology appears nearly unchanged after

Table 4.2 Treatment of osteo-cartilage fragments

Osteosynthesis with screws	Hämmerle and Jacob (1980); Lange et al. (1986); Myllynen et al. (1986); Rae and Khasawneh (1988); McNamee et al. (1988); Gerard et al. (1989); Benedetto et al. (1980); Lewis and Foster (1990)
Wire suturing	Rees and Thompson (1985)
PGA pin fixation	Weh et al. (1982); Lutten et al. (1988); Kristensen et al. (1990)
Fibrin glue	Meyers and Herron (1984); Zilch und Talke (1987); Schlag and Redl (1988); Lutten et al. (1988); Visuri and Kuusela (1989); Angermann and Riegels-Nielsen (1990)
Conservative treatment with plaster of Paris	Dutkowsky and Freeman (1989)
Bone pegs	Hämmerle and Jacob (1980); Baudenbacher and Ricklin (1983); Myllynen et al. (1986)
Homologous grafts	Gross et al. (1983); Kusnick et al. (1987)

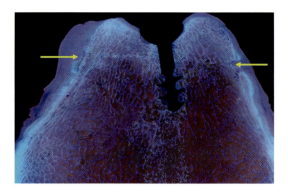

Fig. 4.7 Healed osteotomy (*arrows*) screwed with adapted AO-screws and related defect in the joint's surface 33 days following the operation. Animal experiment on shepherd dogs (Garde 1995) with standardized osteo-cartilage fragment through the condyles of the patellar groove, screwed and dowelled with plugs taken from the transition zone; fresh cross section through the distal femur. Horizontal field width=42 mm. Documentation in the HIIFL microscope in UV-light (ZOW)

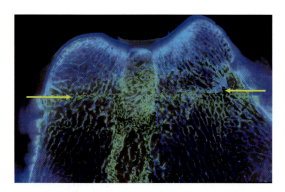

Fig. 4.6 Cross section of an osteocartilage osteotomy fragment (*arrows*), dowelled with two autologous cartilage-bone grafts. Twenty-seven days after the operation, the osteotomy has healed. The press-fit dowel reveals the *yellow label* of the first and second weeks. Contact healing of all cancellous structures is presented. Animal experiment on shepherd dogs (Garde 1995) with standardized osteocartilage fragment through the condyles of the patellar groove, screwed and dowelled plugs taken from the transition zone; fresh, cross section through the distal femur. Horizontal field width=42 mm. Documentation in the HIIFL microscope in UV-light (ZOW)

3 months, the suture line of the cartilage has disappeared (Fig. 4.12), and after 1 year, no difference to the epiphyseal recipient bed can be observed (Fig. 4.13).

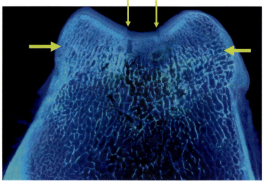

Fig. 4.8 Healed osteotomized cartilage-bone fragment after 1 year in the animal experiment (Garde 1995): the hyaline cartilage, as well as all cancellous bone trabeculae, has healed primarily (*arrows*). A healing ad integrum is pronounced. Fresh cross section through the distal femur. Horizontal field width=42 mm. Documentation in the HIIFL microscope in UV-light (ZOW)

4.3 Metaphyseal Bone

The first milestone on the road to the modern view of bone healing was when Du Hamel (1739) brought Galen's doctrine of "gluing liquids" to an end. Dupuytren (1820) recognized the importance of the provisional callus for the restriction of movements of the fracture ends and defined the definitive callus.

4.3 Metaphyseal Bone

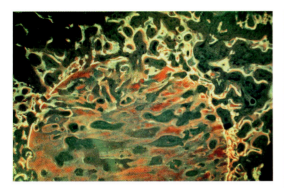

Fig. 4.9 Press-fit inserted autologous graft from the epiphysis revealing bony ingrowth and contact healing after 8 days. There is bony ingrowth of 1,500 μm measured with the labeled new bone formation. MMA-embedded cross section of a rabbit's distal femur; alkaline fuchsine staining. Horizontal field width=6 mm. Leitz Orthoplan; Apochromat 10× Oil, incident fluorescent light, Ploemopak FITC filter system

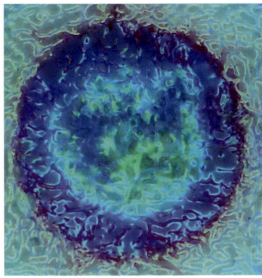

Fig. 4.11 Press-fit inserted bone graft (9.55 mm) in the distal femur of a minipig (Schnettler 1992), 33 days after implantation. There is complete primary contact healing marked. The sequence of labels is *yellow*, followed by *red*, *blue*, and *green* labeling. Fresh cross section in the HIIFL microscope of the ZOW. Horizontal field width=12 mm

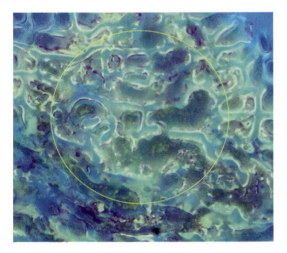

Fig. 4.10 Press-fit inserted autologous graft (*circle*) from the epiphysis revealing bony integration and contact healing after 4 weeks. There is bony integration labeled with tetracycline (*yellow*) and Alizarin complexone (*red*). MMA embedded cross-section of a rabbit's distal femur; alkaline fuchsine staining. Horizontal field width=7 mm. Leitz Orthoplan, incident fluorescent light, Apochromat 10× Oil, Ploemopak UV filter system

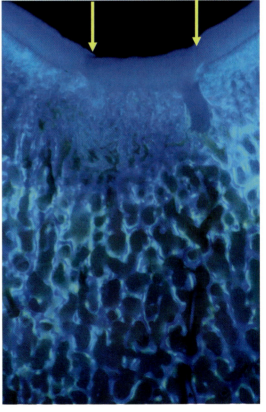

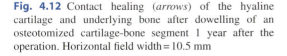

Fig. 4.12 Contact healing (*arrows*) of the hyaline cartilage and underlying bone after dowelling of an osteotomized cartilage-bone segment 1 year after the operation. Horizontal field width=10.5 mm

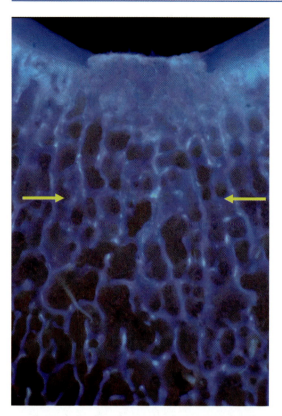

Fig. 4.13 Healing of the cancellous bone (*arrows*) of the epiphysis after osteocartilage osteotomy 1 year after intervention with autologous cartilage-bone dowels. The cartilage is destroyed by direct insertion using pusher and hammer without shear protection of the applicator tube. Horizontal field width = 10.5 mm

John Hunter (1798) discovered resorption on the fracture ends, with which Ollier (1867) completed his description of spontaneous bone healing; he used the term "action de présence." Sixty years later, König (1927) defined resorption on the fracture ends as a specific response of bone to trauma.

Bier's interpretation of the hematoma between the fracture ends (1917) correlates to Lexer's hyperemia around the fracture gap (1936). Virchow's doctrine of metaplasia (1884), Axhausen's teaching of the osteoblasts (1908a, b), and Hintsche's (1927) conclusion regarding the osteoblast doctrine, together with Lubarsch's (1930) formulation of the indirect metaplasia, provided the basis for the theory of differentiation of the pluripotential mesenchyme which made the BMP discovery (Urist et al. 1967) possible.

Voetsch (1847) was the first to mention the concept of "primary and secondary bone healing" in relation to spontaneous and delayed healing. Lane (1914) applied it as well to the question of whether callus formation is pronounced or not. Ultimately, it was Krompecher (1934) who worked out the histopathology of the strain-adapted differentiation of the pluripotential mesenchyme. He introduced the term "primary angiogenetic bone formation" in the case where there is no temporary formation of connective tissue.

Pauwels (1940, 1960) defined the specific stimulus for the differentiation of the pluripotential mesenchymal cell by its deformation and change in volume. Perren and Cordey (1977) and Perren and Boitzy (1978) developed the concept of the relative deformation of the cell, for which doctrine Wurmbach (1928) and Altmann (1950), together with Krompecher (1934), had already delivered the morphological substrate.

Matzen (1952) and (1954) presented the direct relationship between interfragmentary compression, stability with respect to relative motion of the fracture ends, and callus formation. Finally, Danis (1949) introduced interfragmentary compression, achieving "une soudure autogène" without callus formation. Wagner (1963) and Schenk and Willenegger (1963) published the histomorphology of primary bone healing.

Charnley (1948) and (1953) succeeded in achieving osteosynthesis with interfragmentary compression for the metaphyseal bone as well. He spoke about the healing activity of the metaphysis as a "very restricted form of osteogenic activity" but changed the load axis in that case. Draenert and Draenert (1979) worked out the histomorphology of cancellous bone healing.

The first phase comprises the formation of woven bone during the first week (Fig. 4.14), followed by the lamellar reinforcement of the second week (Fig. 4.15) and temporarily finalized by the conversion to compact bone during the third week (Fig. 4.16). From that time, remodeling starts and reaches a final stage after 12 weeks (Fig. 4.17). Contact healing could only be achieved by press-fit insertion of cancellous bone cylinders gathered by means of a wet-grinding process using twin diamond instruments. Complete healing within 4 weeks depended on the diameter of the graft (Fig. 4.18). As opposed to contact healing, defects in cancellous bone do not heal (Figs. 4.19 and 4.20).

4.3 Metaphyseal Bone

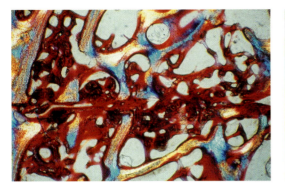

Fig. 4.14 Woven bone framework in a beagle's tibial head 8 days after a hemiosteotomy. Primary metaphyseal bone healing is presented. MMA-embedded cross section in polarized light. Horizontal field width=5.2 mm. Leitz Orthoplan. Apochromat 2.5×

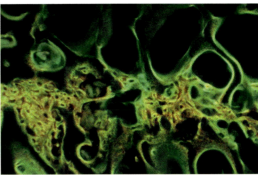

Fig. 4.16 Conversion to compact bone at the end of the third week in a beagle's tibial head after hemiosteotomy and osteosynthesis. Primary metaphyseal bone healing is marked; the reinforcement of the scaffold is labeled with tetracycline (*yellow*). MMA-embedded cross section in incident fluorescent light. Horizontal field width=5.2 mm. Leitz Orthoplan. Ploemopak FITC filter system; Apochromat 2.5×

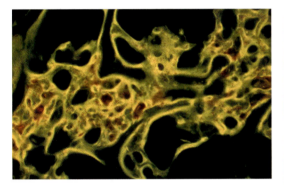

Fig. 4.15 Lamellar reinforcement of the woven bone framework in a beagle's tibial head, 2 weeks after hemiosteotomy and osteosynthesis. Primary metaphyseal bone healing is pronounced. The reinforcement of the scaffold is labeled with tetracycline (*yellow*). Horizontal field width=5.2 mm. MMA-embedded cross section in incident fluorescent light. Leitz Orthoplan. Ploemopak FITC filter-system; Apochromat 2.5×

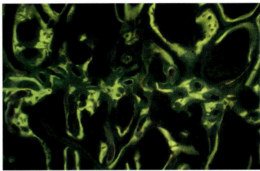

Fig. 4.17 Remodeling stage after 12 weeks in a beagle's tibial head after hemiosteotomy and osteosynthesis. There is primary metaphyseal bone healing marked with restitutio ad integrum; the reinforcement of the scaffold is labeled with tetracycline (*yellow*). MMA-embedded cross section in incident fluorescent light. Horizontal field width=5.2 mm. Leitz Orthoplan. Ploemopak FITC filter system; Apochromat 2.5×

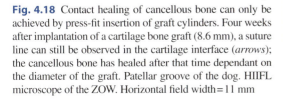

Fig. 4.18 Contact healing of cancellous bone can only be achieved by press-fit insertion of graft cylinders. Four weeks after implantation of a cartilage bone graft (8.6 mm), a suture line can still be observed in the cartilage interface (*arrows*); the cancellous bone has healed after that time dependant on the diameter of the graft. Patellar groove of the dog. HIIFL microscope of the ZOW. Horizontal field width=11 mm

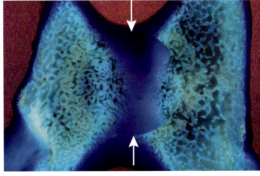

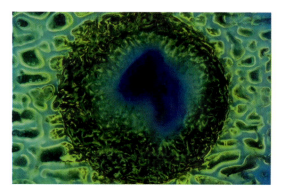

Fig. 4.19 Defect in the patellar groove of a rabbit, measuring 5.4 mm, 4 weeks after the operation. A funnel-shaped healing pattern is pronounced and labeled with *yellow, red*, and *green* fluorochromes. There is still an open connection to the medullary cavity. Epiphyseal defects do not heal ad integrum. MMA-embedded cross section in incident fluorescent light. Horizontal field width = 7.8 mm. Leitz Orthoplan. Ploemopak FITC filter system; Apochromat 4×

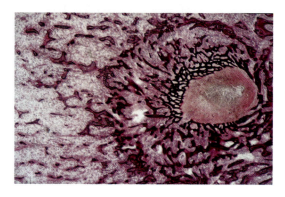

Fig. 4.20 Defect in the metaphysis of a dog measuring 5.4 mm: incomplete healing with funnel-shaped deformation of the defect 4 weeks after the operation. MMA-embedded cross section in transmitted light. Horizontal field width = 7.8 mm. Leitz Orthoplan: Apochromat 4×

There are no studies known in which the cancellous bone healing was combined with BMP 2 or BMP 7; in recent studies, it was reported that sclerostin antibody treatment enhances the metaphyseal bone healing tremendously (Agholme et al. 2010).

References

Agholme F, Li X, Isaksson H et al (2010) Sclerostin antibody treatment enhances metaphyseal bone healing in rats. J Bone Miner Res 25:2412–2418

Altmann K (1950) Untersuchungen über Frakturheilung unter besonderen experimentellen Bedingungen. Z Anat Entwicklungsges 115:52–81

Angermann P, Riegels-Nielsen P (1990) Fibrin fixation of osteochondral talar fracture. Acta Orthop Scand 61:551–553

Axhausen G (1908a) Histologische Untersuchungen über Knochentransplantationen am Menschen. Dtsch Z Chir 91:388–428

Axhausen G (1908b) Die pathologisch-anatomischen Grundlagen der Lehre von der freien Knochentransplantation beim Menschen und Tier. Med klin Beihefte 2:23

Bachelin P, Bugmann P (1988) Active subluxation in extension radiological control in intercondylar eminence fractures in childhood. Z Kinderchir 43:180–182

Barber FA, Prudich JF (1993) Acute traumatic knee hemarthrosis. Arthroscopy 9:174–176

Baudenbacher R, Ricklin P (1983) Knochenspanbolzung bei osteochondralen Kleinfragfrakturen und Osteochondrosis dissecans. Helv Chir Acta 50:655–661

Benedetto KP, Sperner G, Glotzer W (1980) Knee joint hemarthrosis – differential diagnostic considerations for planning an operation. Orthopaede 19:69–76

Berndt AL, Harty M (1959) Transchondral fractures (osteochondritis dissecans) of the talus. J Bone Joint Surg 41-A:988–1020

Bier A (1917) Über Knochenregeneration über Pseudarthrosen und Knochentransplantate. Arch Klin Chir 127:1–136

Blasier RB, Burkus JK (1988) Management of the posterior fracture-dislocations of the shoulder. Clin Orthop 232:197–204

Bohart PG, Gelbermann RH, Vandell RF et al (1982) Complex dislocations of the metacarpophalangeal joint. Clin Orthop 164:208–225

Bomberg BC, McGinty JB (1990) Acute hemarthrosis of the knee: indications for diagnostic arthroscopy. Arthroscopy 6:221–225

Butler JC, Andrews JR (1988) The role of arthroscopic surgery in the evaluation of acute traumatic hemarthrosis of the knee. Clin Orthop 228:150–152

Charnley J (1948) Positive pressure in arthrodesis of the knee joint. J Bone Joint Surg 30-B:478–486

Charnley J (1953) Compression arthrodesis; including central dislocation as a principle in hip surgery. Livingstone, Edinburgh

Danis R (1949) Théorie et pratique de l'ostéosynthèse. Masson, Paris

Dell'accio F, Vincent TL (2010) Joint surface defects: clinical corse and cellular response in spontaneous and experimental lesions. Eur Cell Mater 20:210–217

Draenert K, Draenert Y (1979) The architecture of metaphyseal bone healing SEM. SEM Inc, O'Hare, pp 521–528

Draenert Y, Draenert K (1981) Histo-Morphologie der Tangentialfaserschicht nach Kreuzbandläsion Eine tierexperimentelle Studie am Kniegelenk der Ratte. In: Jäger M Hackenbroch MH, Refior HJ (eds) Kapselbandläsionen des Kniegelenkes. Georg Thieme, Stuttgart, pp 88–92

Draenert ME (2012) "Drug Delivery"- Systeme für den Knochenaufbau. Experimentelle Studie als Grundlage für die Augmentation der Kieferknochen in der Parodontologie. Habilitationsschrift an der Ludwig-Maximilians Universität München

References

Du Hamel HL (1739) Sur une racine qui a la faculté de teindre en rouge les os des animaux vivants. Mém de Mathématique et de Physique de l'Académie Royale des Sciences, Paris, pp 1–13

Dupuytren G (1820) Exposé de la doctrine de M le Professeur Dupuytren sur le cal. Par Samson L J J des Sciences méd. Masson, Paris

Dutkowsky J, Freeman BL (1989) Fracture-dislocation of the articular surface of the third metatarsal head. Foot Ankle 10:43–44

Feder KS, Schonholtz GJ (1992) Ankle arthroscopy: review and long-term results of the talus. J Foot Surg 31:134–140

Frank A, Cohen P, Beaufils P et al (1989) Arthroscopic treatment of osteochondral lesions of the talar dome. Arthroscopy 5:57–61

Frenkel SR, Saadeh PB, Mehrara BJ et al (2000) Transforming growth factor beta superfamily members: role in cartilage modeling. Plast Reconstr Surg 105:980–990

Garde U (1995) Histomorphologie der primären Knochenheilung der Osteochondralfraktur. Die knöchernen Umbauvorgänge und restitutio ad integrum im Tierexperiment. Habilitationsschrift Universität, Trnava

Gerard Y, Bernier JM, Ameil M (1989) Osteochondral lesions of the talus. Rev Chir Orthop 75:466–478

Gilbert TJ, Johnson E, Detlie T et al (1993) Radiologic case study patellar dislocation: medial retinacular tears avulsion fractures and osteochondral fragments. Orthopaedics 16:732–736

Gilley JS, Gelman MI, Edson DM et al (1981) Chondral fractures of the knee. Arthrographic arthroscopic and clinical manifestations. Radiology 138:51–54

Green DP, O'Brien ET (1980) Classification and management of carpal dislocations. Clin Orthop 149:55–72

Gross AE, McKee NH, Pritzker KP et al (1983) Reconstruction of skeletal deficits at the knee. A comprehensive osteochondral transplant program. Clin Orthop 174:96–106

Hämmerle CP, Jacob RP (1980) Chondral and osteochondral fractures after luxation of the patella and their treatment. Arch Orthop Trauma Surg 97:207–211

Hardaker WJ Jr, Garrett WE Jr, Bassett FH (1990) Evaluation of acute traumatic hemarthrosis of the knee joint. South Med J 83:640–644

Hintsche E (1927) Untersuchungen an Stützgeweben. I Teil: Über die Bedeutung der Gefässkanäle im Knorpel und Befunden am distalen Ende des menschlichen Schenkelbeines. Z Mikrosk Anat Forsch 12:61–126

Holzheimer R, Kunze K (1987) Osteochondral fracture in the area of the ankle joint. Unfallchir 13:223–224

Hontas MJ, Haddad RJ, Schlesinger LC (1986) Conditions of the talus in the runner. Am J Sports Med 14:486–490

Hunter J (1798) Experiments and observations on the growth of bones. In: Palmer JF (1835) The works of John Hunter FR. Longman Rees Orme Brown Green and Longman, London, pp 315–318

Huylebroek JF, Martens M, Simon JP (1985) Transchondral talar dome fracture. Arch Orthop Trauma Surg 104:238–241

Isaacs CL, Schreiber FC (1992) Patellar osteochondral fracture: the unforeseen hazard of golf. Am J Sorts Med 16:29–38

Jones P (1987) Fatigue failure osteochondral fracture of the proximal phalanx of the great toe. Am J Sports Med 16:616–618

Karlsson C, Lindahl A (2009) Articular cartilage stem cell signaling. Arthritis Res Ther 11:121

Keller J, Andreassen TT, Joyce F et al (1985) Fixation of osteochondral fractures Fibrin sealant tested in dogs. Acta Orthop Scand 56:323–326

Kenny CH (1981) Inverted osteochondral fracture of the talus diagnosed by tomography. J Bone Joint Surg 63-A:1020–1021

König F (1927) Über den Abbau an gebrochenen Knochen, Sein Wesen und seine Bedeutung. Arch klin Chir 146:624–643

Kristensen G, Lind T, Lavard P et al (1990) Fracture stage 4 of the lateral talar dome treated arthroscopically using Biofix for fixation. Arthroscopy 6:242–244

Krompecher St (1934) Die Entwicklung der Knochenzellen und die Bildung der Knochengrundsubstanz bei der knorpelig und bindegewebig vorgebildeten sowie der primär reinen Knochenbildung Verh Anat Ges Würzburg pp 34–38

Kusnick C, Hayward I, Sartoris DJ et al (1987) Radiographic evaluation of joints resurfaced with osteochondral shell allografts. Am J Roentgenol 149:743–748

Lane WA (1914) The operative treatment of fractures, 2nd edn. The Publishing Cy, London

Lange RH, Engber WD, Clancy WG (1986) Expanding applications for the Herbert scaphoid screw. Orthopaedics 9:1393–1397

Laredo JD, Bellaiche L, Hamze B (1993) The role of MRI of the knee. Ann Radiol 36:200–206

Larson B, Light TR, Ogden JA (1987) Fracture and ischemic necrosis of the immature scaphoid. J Hand Surg (Am) 12:122–127

Lewis PL, Foster BK (1990) Herbert screw fixation of osteochondral fractures about the knee. Austr N Z J Surg 60:511–513

Lexer E (1936) Der Einfluss der Sympathikusunterbrechung auf die Knochenbruchheilung im Tierversuch. Arch Klin Chir 186:242–243

Light TR, Ogden JA (1988) Complex dislocation of the index metacarpophalangeal joint in children. J Pediatr Orthop 8:300–305

Lubarsch O (1930) Zur Lehre von der Metaplasie. Dtsch Z Chir 227:48

Lutten C, Lorenz H, Thomas W (1988) Refixation bei der Osteochondrosis dissecans mit resorbierbarem Material unter Verlaufsbeobachtung mit der Kernspintomographie (MR). Sportverletz Sportschaden 2:61–68

Maquire JK, Canale ST (1993) Fractures of the patella in children and adolescents. J Pediatr Orthop 13:567–571

Matzen PF (1952) Vom Einfluss mechanischer Einwirkungen auf die Kallusbildung. I Teil. Bruns Beitr Klin Chir 184:147–179

Matzen PF (1954) Vom Einfluss mechanischer Einwirkungen auf die Kallusbildung. II Teil. Bruns Beitr Klin Chir 188:97–108

Mazel C, Rigault P, Padovani JP et al (1986) Fractures of the talus in children. Apropos of 23 cases. Rev Chir Orthop Reparatrice 72:183–195

McElfresh EC, Dobyns JH (1983) Intra-articular metacarpal head fractures. J Hand Surg 8(4):383–393

McNamee PB, Bunker TD, Scott TD (1988) The Herbert screw for osteochondral fractures. J Bone Joint Surg 70-B:145–146

Meyers MH, Herron M (1984) A fibrin adhesive seal for the repair of osteochondral fracture fragments. Clin Orthop 182:258–263

Miligram JW (1985) Case report: osteochondral fracture of the right patella without an osteochondral defect. Skeletal Radiol 14:231–234

Mink JH, Deutsch AL (1989) Occult cartilage and bone injuries of the knee: detection classification and assessment with MR imaging. Radiology 170:823–829

Myllynen P, Alberty-Ryoppy A, Harilainen A (1986) Cortical bone pegs in the treatment of osteochondral fracture of the knee. Ann Chir Gynaecol 75:160–163

Noyes FR, Paulos L, Mooar LA et al (1980) Knee sprains and acute knee hemarthrosis: misdiagnosis of anterior cruciate ligament tears. Phys Ther 60:1596–1601

Ollier L (1867) Traité expérimentale et clinique de la régénération des os et de la production artificielle du tissu osseux. Masson, Paris

Otsuki S, Grogan SP, Miyaki S et al (2010) Tissue neogenesis and STRO-1 expression in immature and mature articular cartilage. J Orthop Res 28:96–102

Ove PN, Bosse MJ, Reinert CM (1989) Excision of posterolateral talar dome lesions through a medial transmalleolar approach. Foot Ankle 9:171–175

Paar O, Boszotta H (1991) Avulsion fractures of the knee and upper ankle joint. Classification and therapy. Chirurg 62:121–125

Parisien JS, Vangsness T (1985) Operative arthroscopy of the ankle. Three year's experience. Clin Orthop 199:46–53

Pauwels F (1940) Grundriss einer Biomechanik der Frakturheilung. Verh Dtsch Orthop Ges 34:62–108

Pauwels F (1960) Eine neue Theorie über den Einfluss mechanischer Reize auf die Differenzierung der Stützgewebe. Z Anat Entwicklungsges 121:478–515

Perren SM, Boitzy A (1978) Cellular differentiation and bone biomechanics during the consolidation of a fracture. Anat Clinica 1:13–28

Perren SM, Cordey J (1977) Die Gewebsdifferenzierung in Frakturheilung. Z Unfallheilk 80:161–164

Pettine KA, Morrey BF (1987) Osteochondral fractures of the talus. A long-term follow-up. J Bone Joint Surg 69-A:89–92

Quintin A, Schizas C, Scaletta C et al (2010) Plasticity of fetal cartilaginous cells. Cell Transplant 19:1349–1357

Rae PS, Khasawneh ZM (1988) Herbert screw fixation of osteochondral fractures of the patella. Injury 19:116–119

Ragnarsson B, Danckwardt-Lilliestrom G, Mjoberg B (1992) The triradiate incision for acetabular fractures. A prospective study of 23 cases. Acta Orthop Scand 63:515–519

Rees W, Thompson SK (1985) Osteochondral fractures of the patella. A method of fixation. J R Coll Surg Edinb 30:88–90

Runow A (1983) The dislocating patella. Etiology and prognosis in relation to generalized joint laxity and anatomy of the patellar articulation. Acta Orthop Scand 201:1–53

Saffar P (1984) Carpal luxation and residual instability. Ann Chir Main 3:349–352

Schenk R, Willenegger H (1963) Zum histologischen Bild der sogenannten Primärheilung der Knochenkompakta nach experimentellen Osteotomien am Hund. Experientia 19:593–595

Schild H, Ahlers J (1987) Traumatology of the knee joint – radiologic and accident surgery aspects. Part 1. Roentgenblätter 40:263–269

Schlag G, Redl H (1988) Fibrin sealant in orthopaedic surgery. Clin Orthop 227:269–285

Schnettler R (1992) Vergleichende Untersuchungen zum Einwachsverhalten von autogenen und allogenen Spongiosatransplantaten im Vergleich zu Keramik, DBM und basischem Fibroblastenwachstumsfaktor (bFGF). Habilitationsschrift. Universität Leipzig

Silberberg M, Silberberg R, Hasler M (1965a) Early effects of somatotropin on the fine structure of articular cartilage. Anat Rec 151:297–314

Silberberg R, Hasler M, Silberberg M (1965b) Submicroscopic response of articular cartilage of mice treated with estrogenic hormone. Am J Path 46:289–305

Stanitski CL, Harvell JC, Fu F (1993) Observations on acute knee hemarthrosis in children and adolescents. J Pediatr Orthop 13:506–510

Stripling WD (1982) Displaced intra-articular osteochondral fracture-cause for irreducible dislocation of the distal interphalangeal joint. J Hand Surg (Am) 7:77–78

Sun J, Hou XK, Kuang Y et al (2011) Influence of the unevenness of articular cartilage surface on the osteochondral repair. Zhongguo Gu Shang 24:505–508

Tehranzadeh J, Vanarthos W, Pais MJ (1990) Osteochondral impaction of the femoral head associated with hip dislocation: CT study in 35 patients. Am J Roentgenol 155:1049–1052

Tokuhara Y, Wakintani S, Imai Y et al (2010) Repair of experimentally induced large osteochondral defects in rabbit knee with various concentrations of *Escherichia coli*-derived recombinant human bone morphogenetic protein-2. Int Orthop 34:761–767

Torg JS, Pavlov H, Morris VB (1981) Salter-Harris type III fracture of the medial femoral condyle occurring in the adolescent athlete. J Bone Joint Surg 63-A:568–591

References

Urist MR, Silverman BF, Buring K et al (1967) The bone induction principle. Clin Orthop 53:243–283

Vellet AD, Marks PH, Fowler PJ et al (1991) Occult post-traumatic osteochondral lesions of the knee: prevalence classification and short-term sequelae evaluated with MR imaging. Radiology 178:271–276

Virchow R (1884) Über Metaplasie. Virchows Arch 97:410

Visuri T, Kuusela T (1989) Fixation of large osteochondral fractures of the patella with fibrin adhesive system. A report of two operative cases. Am J Sports Med 17:842–845

Voetsch A (1847) Die Heilung der Knochenbrüche per primam intentionem. Winter, Heidelberg

Wagner H (1963) Die Einbettung von Metallschrauben im Knochen und die Heilungsvorgänge des Knochengewebes unter dem Einfluss der stabilen Osteosynthese. Langenbecks Arch klin Chir 305:28–41

Wasilewski SA, Frankl U (1992) Osteochondral avulsion fracture of femoral insertion of anterior cruciate ligament. Case report and review of literature. Am J Sports Med 20:224–226

Weh L, Korn U, Dahmen G (1982) Freie Gelenkkörper im Kniegelenk. Ätiologie, Klinik und therapeutisches Konzept. Fortschr Med 100:1939–1943

Wertheimer SJ, Balzsy JE (1992) A unique osteochondral fracture of the first metatarsophalangeal joint. J Foot Surg 31:49–67

Wilson WJ, Scranton PE Jr (1990) Combined reconstruction of the anterior cruciate ligament in competitive athletes. J Bone Joint Surg 72-A:742–748

Wurmbach H (1928) Histologische Untersuchungen über die Heilung von Knochenbrüchen bei Säugern. Z Zool 132:200–256

Zilch H, Talke M (1987) Fibrogen glue in osteochondral fractures with small fragments of the upper limb. Ann Chir Main 6:173–176

Ceramic Bone Substitutes 5

5.1 Bioglasses

Bioglasses represent noncrystalline compositions which are normally mélanges of alkaline and acid oxides. Alkaline oxides are Na, K, Mg, Ca, or Ba oxides, whereas silicium dioxide represents a well-known molecule for reticulations. Bioglasses are used in coating implants (Hench et al. 1971). Since the manufacturing processes of physiological calcium phosphates have been improved enormously, bioglasses play no role in bone substitution at the moment.

5.2 Ceramics

Aluminum silicates, natural earths, sintered at high temperature, represent the original materials known as ceramics. Today, ceramics cover a wide range of products; the nature of all ceramics is inorganic, nonmetallic materials, treated by heat. As bone void fillers or as bone substitutes, the physiological calcium phosphates comprise ß-tricalcium phosphate and hydroxyapatite. Both materials are considered to be biocompatible materials. According to the FDA, those materials are considered medical device products, which implies that there is no local or systemic toxic reaction, no foreign body response, and also no cancerogenicity (Bauer and Smith 2002).

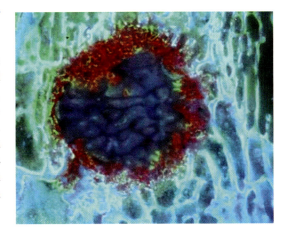

Fig. 5.1 Anisotropic structure of a bovine ceramic 4 weeks after implantation in the distal femur of a rabbit. There is pronounced directed osteoconduction according to the architecture of the bovine ceramic. Documentation in the HIIFL microscope in UV-light (ZOW): the *yellow*, *red*, and *green labels* are well pronounced. Horizontal field width = 7.8 mm

5.2.1 Bovine Ceramics

Bovine ceramics are processed and ultimately sintered from bovine cancellous bone gathered mainly from the metaphysis. Blocs and cylinders represent stiff, strong, and brittle scaffolds of the bovine bone revealing an anisotropic structure (Fig. 5.1). The granulated material reveals nearly compact material. The implants consist of 95% hydroxyapatite. Their compressive strength depends on their anisotropic structure and differs greatly according

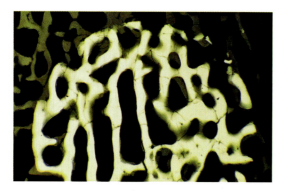

Fig. 5.2 Delicate bony ingrowth crossing the interface of a bovine ceramic 22 months after implantation in the patellar groove of a rabbit. The stiff implant yields stress protection inside the ceramic scaffold. Microradiograph of a 60-µm-thick cross section. Horizontal field width = 6.31 mm

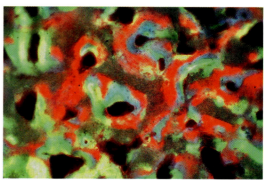

Fig. 5.4 Ceramic-reinforced bone 6 weeks after implantation in a 4.6 mm defect of a rabbit's patellar groove. The sequence of labels is *yellow, red, blue*, and *green* continuously applied over 35 days, starting with the fifth day. The sandwich formation represents new ceramic-bone material. Cross section is stained with basic fuchsine in the Orthoplan (Leitz) with Ploemopak and UV-filter system. Apochromat 10×, Oil. Horizontal field width = 1.0 mm

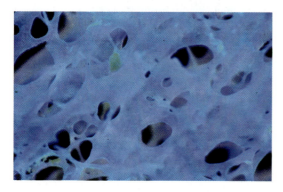

Fig. 5.3 Shell-like cancellous bone in the tibial head of a 12-year-old boy. Incident fluorescent light (*dark field*). Leitz Makrozoom. Horizontal width field = 3.1 mm

5.2.2 Coralliform Ceramics

Hydroxyapatite (HA) implants are also processed in the laboratory from corals; the coralliform calcium carbonate is transferred to HA through a so-called replaminiform process (White et al. 1972; White and Shors 1986; Holmes et al. 1988). The pores of those implants are smaller than pores in the bovine ceramic implants; the architecture is more uniform and the trabeculae are thick and compact.

5.2.3 Synthetic Ceramics – HA and ß-TCP

All bone substitutes available on the market offer a structure which imitates or reproduces the physiological structure of bone. These implants can be described as "positively" structured or "sandwich former" because, overgrown on both sides by newly formed bone, they reveal a bone–ceramic–bone sandwich (Fig. 5.4). Cancellous bone was called by anatomists "shell" bone (Weidenreich 1923) in the early literature and can be synthetically manufactured as HA, as well as ß-TCP implant and in a completely interconnected form (Fig. 5.5a, b), thus providing the

to the correspondence of the axis of the cattle bone to the structure of the implant under load (Draenert et al. 2001). Stiff implants transfer the load acting on them directly to the underlying bone, thus serving as a cavity shield. Bony ingrowth occurs only after microfracturing of the trabeculae due to cyclic loading. The bone grows into the implant with its strong and compact trabeculae (Fig. 5.2). On the other hand, colonization by osteoblasts and bony ingrowth relates directly to the specific surface area, that is the surface area per cubic centimeter of the implant, impressively documented in juvenile bone that is a shell in its natural state (Fig. 5.3).

5.3 Chemistry of Calcium Phosphates

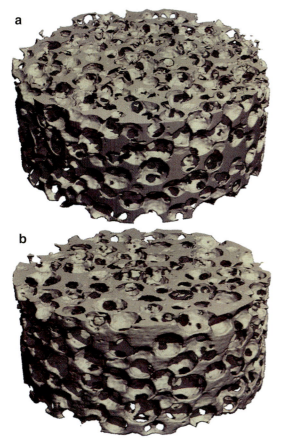

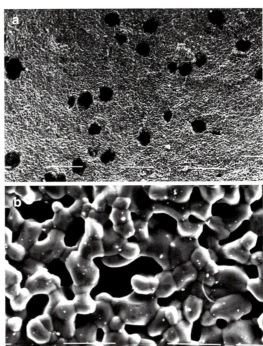

Fig. 5.6 (**a**) SEM of the Synthacer® surface revealing micropores of about 30–50 μm. Horizontal field width = 700 μm. (**b**) High resolution in the SEM of the HA surface. The nanopores measure 5–10 μm. Horizontal field width = 50 μm

Fig. 5.5 (**a**) μ-CT of a synthetic HA implant (Synthacer®). The macropores comprise 600 μm. Horizontal field width = 8.4 mm. (**b**) μ-CT of a synthetic ß-TCP implant (Syntricer®). The macropores measure 600 μm. Horizontal field width = 8.4 mm

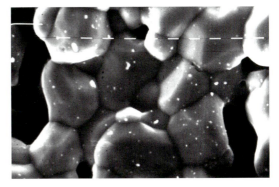

Fig. 5.7 Sintered crystallites in the SEM. There is an even structure of the sintered crystallites measuring between 3 and 5 μm. Horizontal field width = 25 μm

highest possible surface per cubic centimeter (ss = specific surface). The ultrastructure of pure synthetically manufactured material is quite uniform (Fig. 5.6a, b) and the microcrystals evenly connected (Fig. 5.7). Synthetic material is highly pure material because the raw material has already been examined for heavy metals or other impurities. The examination is conducted using an X-ray diffractogram (Fig. 5.8), chemical analysis, and measuring compressive strengths (Fig. 5.9).

A new injection molding process allows for the manufacturing of strong implants of both materials, HA and ß-TCP, providing 80–85% porosity (Figs. 5.10a, b and 5.11a, b).

5.3 Chemistry of Calcium Phosphates

Bone contains a certain amount of tricalcium phosphate. The formula is $Ca_3(PO_4)_2$ (TCP). The ratio of calcium to phosphate is 1.5:1. There are

Fig. 5.8 X-ray diffractograph of Synthacer® identified according to the ICDD (International Center for Diffraction Data = former JCPDS, Joint Committee on Powder Diffraction Standards)

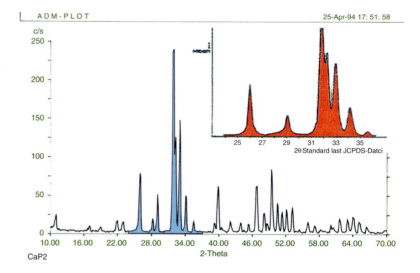

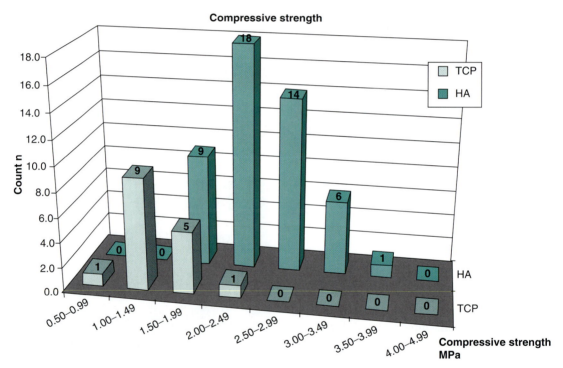

Fig. 5.9 Compressive strength of ß-TCP (Syntricer®) compared with HA (Synthacer®)

two different crystal lattices: the low-temperature complex of ß-Whitlockit structure and the more stable α-Whitlockit structure that forms at temperatures of over 1,300°C.

Hydroxyapatite is a pentacalcium hydroxytriphosphate: $Ca_5(PO_4)_3OH = Ca_{10}(PO_4)_6(OH)_2$. The ratio of calcium and phosphate is 1.67:1. Hydroxyapatite is the main mineral component of bone and comprises 90% and more. The hardness of the material according to Moh is five. Hydroxyapatite has a hexagonal dipyramidal crystal lattice, and its density makes up 3 g per ccm. The lattice structure is measured via X-ray diffractometry and is listed under the JCPDS standards (Joint Committee on Powdered Diffraction Standards, ICDD = International Center for Diffraction Data).

Fig. 5.10 (**a**) HA Synthacer® implant. Diameter of the cylinder = 6.35 mm. (**b**) NSSC implant "Ceraspine"®, a net-shaped sintered ceramic providing high-level material strength combined with high porosity. Horizontal field width = 7.6 mm

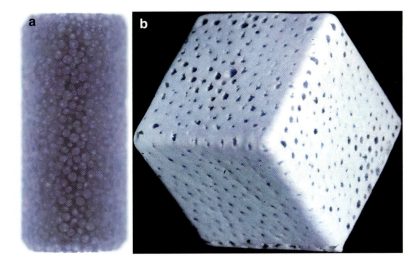

Fig. 5.11 (**a**) ß-TCP Syntricer® implant (6.35 mm). (**b**) NSSC ß-TCP implant comprising up to 85% porosity with high-level material strength. Horizontal field width = 23 mm

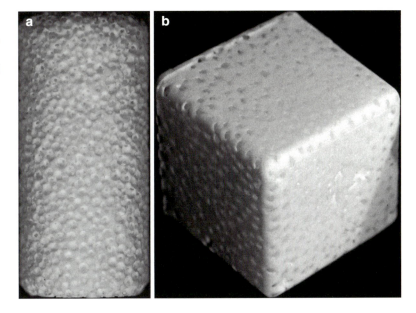

5.4 Osseoconduction – Bony Ingrowth

The osseointegration or osteointegration was introduced as a term for a fibrous-tissue-free implant-to-bone interface (Brånemark et al. 1977; Osborn 1985). The stability of the fixation of ceramic implants plays a major role for its rapid integration. The ceramic implants have to be inserted in a press-fit manner resisting bone deformation. The material should be chosen according to the deformation of the bony bed: HA press-fit cylinders are required for the iliac crest, resisting the pronounced deformation of the iliac crest by the oblique and transverse abdominal muscles (Fig. 5.12). A similar indication is valid for defects in the tibial head, the heel bone, and others for adjuvant fracture treatment. In addition to the osteoconductive function, the high capillary forces of the ceramics provide stop bleeding and carry bone marrow cells for fast regeneration as shown in the femoral condyle (Fig. 5.13).

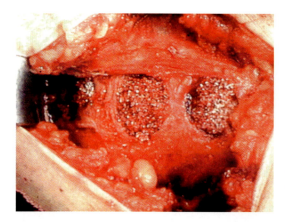

Fig. 5.12 HA press-fit implants (Synthacer®) in precise wet ground defects of the iliac crest avoid donor bed morbidity. The ceramic measures 5/100 mm more than the diameter of the defect. Horizontal field width = 58 mm

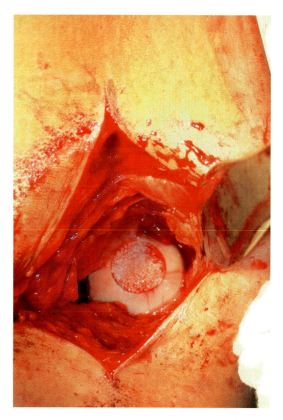

Fig. 5.13 Press-fit ß-TCP implants (Syntricer®) in the posterior distal femoral condyle do not need a cambium tissue providing sling properties. Horizontal field width = 92 mm

Pore sizes of 600 μm with wider interconnections allow for fast sandwich formation and bony integration providing an integrated scaffold of *ceramic reinforced bone*. As far as HA implants are concerned, the construction will become part of the bony scaffold. The discussion about pore sizes is still ongoing (Draenert et al. 2011). The recommendations range from 50–100 μm (Eggli et al. 1988) to 500–600 μm (Kühne et al. 1994; Wiese 1998). It was shown, however, that bone grows into the smallest pores as soon as vascularization is adjacent (Fig. 5.14a). Large implants need reasonable interconnecting openings of not less than 30–50 μm for revascularization (Fig. 5.14b). A reasonable "bone–ceramic–bone" architecture occurs with pore sizes of 500–600 μm in the metaphysis and 300 μm in the epiphysis (Fig. 5.15a, b). In addition, bone ingrowth increases directly proportional to the specific surface of the ceramic (surface per ccm). Shell-like ceramics such as Synthacer® and Syntricer® (Fig. 5.16a–c) provide the largest possible surface combined with high material strength.

The bony integration of both ceramics is completed depending on the diameter of the implant up to 8.35 mm within 4 weeks (Fig. 5.17). The ß-TCP is quickly overgrown with newly formed bone at an even faster rate than HA. ß-TCP is not as stiff as HA (Draenert 2011a).

5.5 Biodegradation

Two different processes, a chemical and a biological one, dissolve calcium phosphate ceramics: the chemical–physical solubility and the degradation of the crystallites by macrophages and multinuclear foreign body giant cells (Draenert 2011a). The chemical, physical dissolution plays no role because ß-TCP and HA are nearly insoluble in water (Renooij et al. 1985). The degradation process is well pronounced in all ß-TCP implants, offering a highly specific surface per ccm (Draenert 2011a). Active resorption by macrophagocytes and multinuclear giant cells represents a complicated process of *remodeling*

5.5 Biodegradation

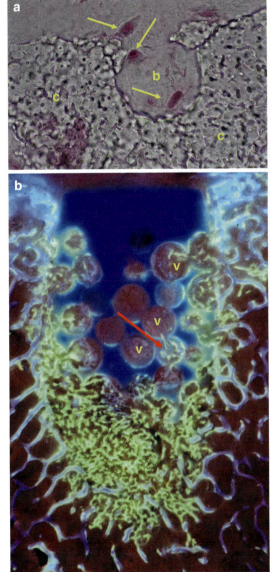

Fig. 5.14 (**a**) Pores along the interface of the ceramic (*c*) measuring less than 50 μm are filled with newly formed bone (*b*) with living osteocytes (*arrows*). Alkaline fuchsine staining. Leitz Orthoplan; Apochromat 63× Oil; 35 μm cross section. Horizontal field width = 300 μm. (**b**) Synthacer® ceramic providing 600-μm pores reveal full revascularization 23 days after the operation, as indicated by the *light blue* fluorescence of the vasculature (*v*). The 600-μm pores provide space for a complete osteon system (*arrow*). Orthoplan (Leitz), Ploemopak, UV-filter. Apochromat 10× Oil. Horizontal field width = 8 mm

resorption: The bone–ceramic–bone sandwich reveals cutter heads of osteoclasts (ceramoclasts, Meiss 1986) in the interface and even in the

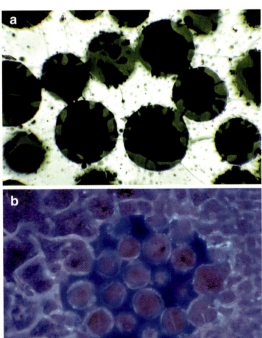

Fig. 5.15 (**a**) Synthacer® implant providing 600-μm pores reveal intact ceramic–bone scaffolding construction 1 year after implantation in the shepherd dog's tibial metaphysis. Microradiograph of a 110-μm-thick MMA-embedded cross section. Leitz Orthoplan. Horizontal field width = 2.4 mm. (**b**) Synthacer® implant providing 300-μm pores in the epiphyseal bone of a dog 1 year after implantation presents a nearly physiological framework of ceramic reinforced bone. HIIFL microscope. Horizontal field width = 3 mm

middle of the ceramic but also along the bony trabeculae (Fig. 5.18). A comparison of ß-TCP and HA over a period of 1 year confirms the reabsorption of ß-TCP within a short time with nearly no absorption of the HA. Osteoclasts, however, can also be found along the HA surface and the path of particles is the same: The phagocyting reticulum cells reveal the intracellular crystals of both (Fig. 5.19a, b). After 1 year, ß-TCP can only be found as intermediate lamella within single trabeculae (Fig. 5.20a, b). The ceramic implant is reabsorbed and a physiological scaffold of newly formed bone is reconstructed (Fig. 5.21a), whereas HA implants became part of the construction (Fig. 5.21b). The direct comparison of

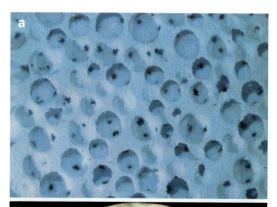
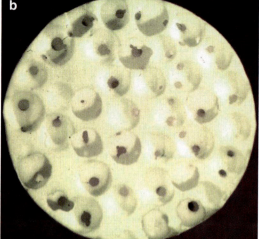
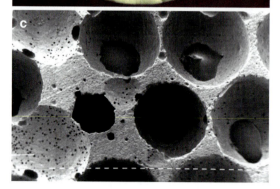
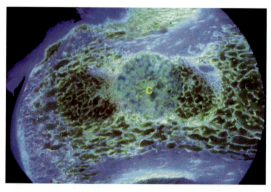

Fig. 5.17 HA Synthacer® ceramic measuring 8.4 mm (*c*) presents complete bony integration in a recipient bed providing damping properties of cancellous bone. The HIIFL microscope was used for documentation in UV-light of a dog's tibial head. Horizontal field width = 29 mm

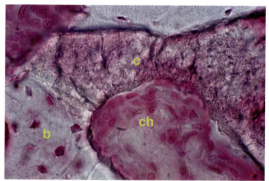

Fig. 5.18 Cutter head (*ch*) of multinuclear giant cells reabsorbing the HA ceramic (*c*) on one side and bone (*b*) on the other. Alkaline fuchsine staining. Leitz Orthoplan, Apochromat 63× Oil. Horizontal field width = 320 μm

Fig. 5.16 (**a**) Shell-like Synthacer® 600 ceramic providing 85% pure HA. Horizontal field width = 5.3 mm. (**b**) Shell-like Syntricer® 300 ceramic that provides at least 85% pure ß-TCP. Horizontal field width = 2.6 mm. (**c**) The shell-like ceramics reveal the highest possible specific surface area for the adherence of the type I collagen fibers. SEM of a cross section of a ceramic with 1,000-μm large pores. Horizontal field width = 2.0 mm

HA and ß-TCP cylinders in the dog tibial head of over a period of 1 year reveals the difference between both materials (Fig. 5.22a–h).

5.6 Granulated Material

Ceramics made of HA or ß-TCP exhibit no osteoinductive effects but are rather exclusively osteoconductive materials which simulate a conductive ladder. In contrast to such osteoconductive scaffolds, granulates are classified as primary non-osteoconductive; they do not give rise to an ordered bone structure (Fig. 5.23) (Draenert et al. 2001). Granulated material should be combined 1:1 with morsellized cancellous bone to

5.6 Granulated Material

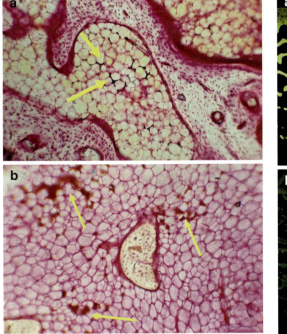

Fig. 5.19 (a) Path of reabsorption of HA crystallites (*arrows*) via the RES. Alkaline fuchsine staining. Cross section of a rabbit's patellar groove recipient bed 2 years after the operation. Horizontal field width = 1.45 mm. (b) Path of reabsorption of ß-TCP crystallites via the RES (*arrows*). Horizontal field width = 1.45 mm

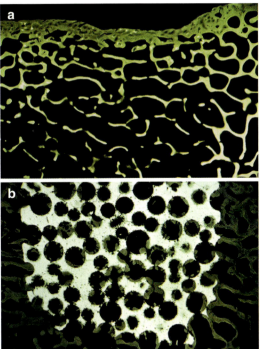

Fig. 5.21 (a) Restitutio ad integrum of a cancellous bone defect 1 year after implantation of a ß-TCP Syntricer® ceramic in the tibial head of a dog. Microradiograph of a 110-μm-thick cross section. Horizontal field width = 6 mm. (b) Incorporation of a HA ceramic (Synthacer®) in the tibial head of a shepherd dog 1 year after implantation. Microradiograph. Horizontal field width = 7.2 mm

avoid fibrous encapsulation or the development of bone cysts – the so-called ceramic disease – due to micromovements (Meiss 1986). The combination of HA-granulated particles and ß-TCP particles with their damping properties allows for implanting a mélange of both directly into defects.

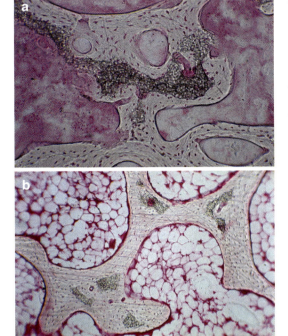

Fig. 5.20 (a) Remodeling resorption of ß-TCP Syntricer® implants in the dog's tibial head 4 months after implantation. Horizontal field width = 1.6 mm. (b) ß-TCP Syntricer® inclusions in a physiological scaffold of cancellous bone 1 year after press-fit insertion in the tibial head of a shepherd dog. Horizontal field width = 1.45 mm

Fig. 5.22 (a–h)
Incorporation and reabsorption of HA and ß-TCP, respectively, over a period of 1 year in the dog experiment. ap X-rays

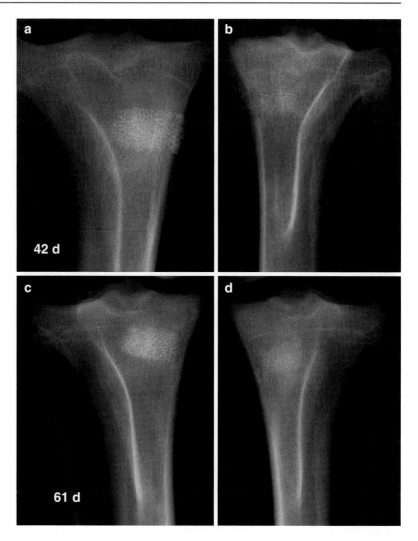

Fig. 5.22 (continued)

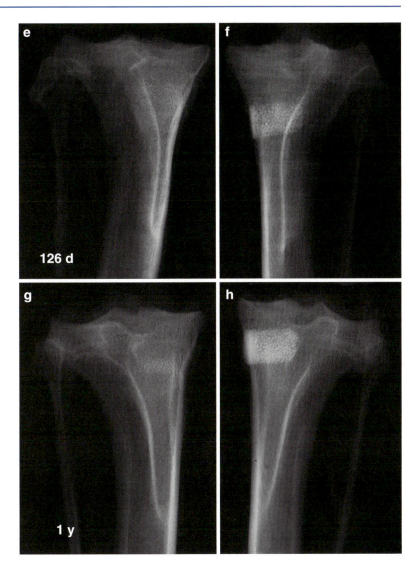

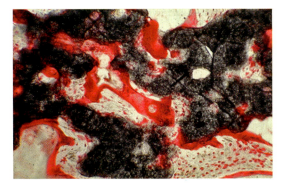

Fig. 5.23 Bony integration of HA (Synthacer®) granulated material in a human biopsy gathered from the tibial head (1y). Despite full osseointegration, a physiological architecture is missing. Alkaline fuchsine staining. Horizontal field width = 1.6 mm

References

Bauer TW, Smith ST (2002) Bioactive materials in orthopaedic surgery: overview and regulatory considerations. Clin Orthop Relat Res 395:11–22

Brånemark PI, Hansson BO, Adell R et al (1977) Osseointegrated implants in the treatment of edontulous jaw. Experience from a 10-year period. Scand J Plast Reconstr Surg Suppl 16:1–132

Draenert AI (2011) Zur Einheilung und Resorption von Hydroxylapatit und ß-Tricalciumphosphat. Eine tierexperimentelle Studie am Tibiakopf des Hundes. Dissertation. Ludwig-Maximilians-Universität München

Draenert K, Wiese FG, Garde U et al (2001) Synthetische Knochenersatzwerkstoffe auf HA- und TCP-Basis. Trauma Berufskrankh 4:293–300

Draenert K, Draenert M, Erler M et al (2011) How bone forms in large cancellous defects: critical analysis based on experimental work and literature. Injury, Int J Care Injured 42:47–55

Eggli PS, Müller W, Schenk RK (1988) Porous hydroxyapatite and tricalcium phosphate cylinders with two different pore size ranges implanted in the cancellous bone of rabbits. A comparative histomorphometric and histologic study of bony ingrowth and implant substitution. Clin Orthop Relat Res 232:127–138

Hench LL, Splinter RJ, Allen T et al (1971) Bonding mechanisms at the interface of ceramic prosthetic materials. J Biomed Mater Res 5:117–141

Holmes RE, Wardrop RW, Wolford LM (1988) Hydroxyapatite as a bone graft substitute in orthognathic surgery: histologic and histometric findings. J Oral Maxillofac Surg 46(8):661–671

Kühne JH, Barti R, Frisch B et al (1994) Bone formation in coralline hydroxyapatite. Effects of pore sized studies in rabbits. Acta Orthop Scand 65:246–252

Meiss L (1986) Untersuchung der Knochenregeneration in standardisierten Knochendefekten des Göttinger Miniaturschweins nach Auffüllung mit zerkleinerten Corticalis und porösen CA-Phosphat Keramiken. Habilitationsschrift der Medizinischen Fakultät, Hamburg

Osborn JF (1985) Die physiologische Integration von Hydroxylapatitkeramiken in das Knochengewebe. Hefte Unfallheilk 174:101–105

Renooij W, Hoogendoorn HA, Visser WJ et al (1985) Bioresorption of ceramic strontium-85-labeled calcium phosphate implants in dog femora. A pilot study to quantitate bioresorption of ceramic implants of hydroxyapatite and tricalcium orthophosphate in vivo. Clin Orthop Relat Res 197:272–285

Weidenreich F (1923) Knochenstudien. 1.Teil: Über Aufbau und Entwicklung des Knochens und den Charakter des Knochengewebes. Z Anat 69:382–466

White E, Shors EC (1986) Biomaterial aspects of Interpore-200 porous hydroxyapatite. Dent Clin North Am 30:49–67

White RA, Weber JN, White NW (1972) Replaminiform: a new process for preparing porous ceramic metal and polymer prosthetic materials. Science 176:922–924

Wiese FG (1998) Histomorphologie einer synthetisch hergestellten Hydroxylapatit ($Ca_5(PO_4)_3OH$) Positivkeramik. Knochenersatzwerkstoff mit reproduzierbarer definierter Porengrösse im interkonnektierenden Porensystem. Dissertation Ludwig-Maximillians-Universität, München

Operating Technique for Cartilage-Bone Grafting

6.1 Basic Principles

For a long time, the Burkhardt's saw-toothed cutter was the only biopsy instrument with which a nearly artifact-free bone cylinder could be gathered (Burkhardt 1956). The first experiments on cancellous bone healing were performed with the low-speed Burkhardt's device. Tissue traumatization in the donor bed, however, was not acceptable for bone healing experiments. Diamond-coated instruments and the wet-grinding procedure had been developed specifically for experiments on the contact healing of cancellous bone (Draenert et al. 1981). Compared with the saw-toothed cutters, nearly no loss of tissue occurred (Fig. 6.1). The technology with respect to cartilage-bone grafts and biopsies (Draenert and Draenert 1987) was ready for application in the early 1980s and publication in 1987. During the evaluation, eight different cutter heads were tested in bovine ribs. As a result, the wet-grinding process using diamond-coated instruments turned out to be the only process to present a nearly atraumatic cylinder and bed, leaving bone and bone marrow of the graft and donor bed intact as well (Fig. 6.1). Those results were published later (Draenert et al. 2007).

The basic principle underlying an atraumatic procedure is the wet-grinding process with an inner rinsing lavage which washes out all debris particles and cools down the heat generated by friction (Fig. 6.2). To preserve the cartilage artifact-free, cartilage, as a soft tissue, has to be cut sharply. The cartilage cutting instrument is integrated into the extractor, providing the sharp edge of the cylindrical tool (Fig. 6.3). Due to its texture, the collagenous tissue opens the gap, thus freeing the bony baseplate for the diamond tool. The hyaline cartilage will be severely damaged yielding a cicatrice if the diamond is used before the sharp extractor has cut the cartilage. With this in mind, the rim of the ground defect presents an absolutely smooth rim.

6.1.1 Basic Guide to Instruments

The diamond tools are coated with natural diamonds, the surface of the metal tool is specially prepared, and the mouth, as well as the inner surface of the tool, is densely covered with sharp diamond particles, ensuring an absolutely precise wall thickness (Fig. 6.4a, b). The diamond grains are electrobonded over two thirds of their surface area and are firmly fixated (Fig. 6.5). In a fatigue test on hard pig bone, the coat was tested, and after 324 procedures, the crown was evaluated in the SEM (Fig. 6.6a, b).

The diamond instrument cuts only hard tissue. It has to be cooled and cleaned by an inner pressure lavage system. In this way, even cortical bone biopsies can be gathered. With the smallest tube comprising diameters of 2.80/3.60 mm, a biopsy of half of the cortex reveals about 150 osteons for evaluation (Fig. 6.7a). The only artifact visible histologically is a slight demineralization along the border up to a depth of 30 μm (Fig. 6.7b).

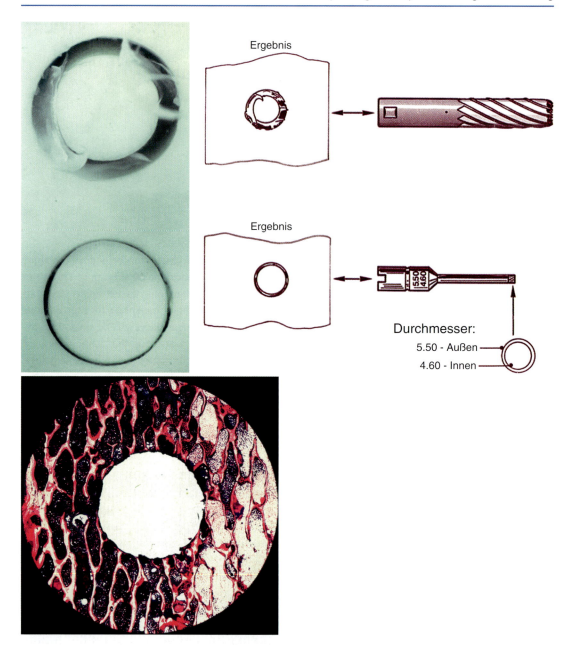

Fig. 6.1 The Burkhardt's myelotomy preserves an intact bone or even cartilage-bone cylinder; however, it severely destroys the donor bed, whereas the wet-grinding diamond tool preserves both, graft and bed. It is a nearly atraumatic procedure, preserving even the bone marrow in the marrow spaces on both sides

In order to obtain a specimen of a biopsy or graft cylinder, a special extractor was designed. For a safe extraction procedure, a precise inner profile comprising three or more barbs arranged to its internal periphery was created by wire erosion combined with a defined roughness of the anterior inner wall of the extractor. The same extractor was prepared with its sharp edge for cutting the cartilage (Fig. 6.8). Pestles with a plastic tip can easily expel the cartilage and bone cores (Fig. 6.9). Precision in operation is ensured by calibration of the diamond grinder and the removal tube (Fig. 6.10a, b).

6.1 Basic Principles

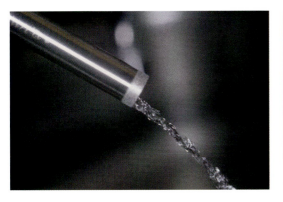

Fig. 6.2 The inner rinsing system is of utmost importance in avoiding heat necrosis and removing wear from the grinding process

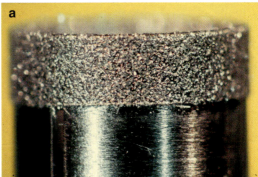

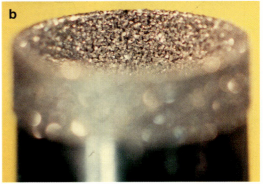

Fig. 6.4 (**a**, **b**) The crown of the grinding tool is coated with natural diamonds. The thickness of the coat is very precise. The rounded end of the tube is also coated

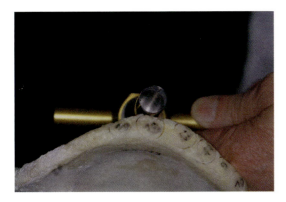

Fig. 6.3 The task for the extractor is twofold: cartilage, as a soft tissue, has to be cut sharply, and the ground cylinder has to be safely twisted off, thus necessitating a precise instrument with an inner profile

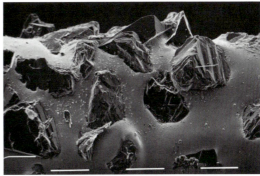

Fig. 6.5 The diamond particles are 60% embedded and safely fixated to the metal tube

6.1.2 Diamond Twins

For transplantation, a press-fit seat of the graft is required. The whole set of diamond instruments is based on the "twins principle": The outer diameter of the smaller tool is 1/10, or 15/100 or even 2/10 mm within the large tools, smaller than the inner diameter of the next following tool (Fig. 6.11).

6.1.3 Irrigation

The internal irrigation system requires a special adapter with an integrated feedline for a physiological solution (NaCl or Ringer). For pressure-feed flushing, an arthroscopic pumping system is suitable. The connections are equipped with a Luer-lock.

The diamond tools are fitted to the adapter of the drill by a quick-action chuck (Fig. 6.12).

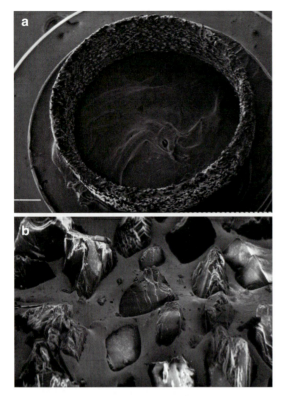

Fig. 6.6 (**a**, **b**) In a fatigue test with more than 300 biopsies gathered from pig bones, the diamond tool was tested and the crown cut and investigated in the SEM. Single diamond particles were cut at the level of the bond. The majority of the circumference, however, showed an intact coat with sharp diamond particles

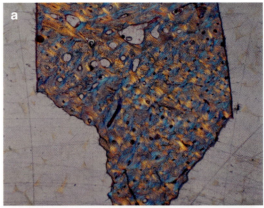

Fig. 6.7 (**a**, **b**) Histology of human cortical biopsies revealed a nearly artifact-free interface of the bone. A slightly demineralized zone up to a depth of 30 μm was the only artifact which could be documented histologically

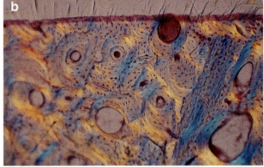

6.1.4 Instrumentation Table

A steritray and a modular instrumentation table provide a clear overview and safe instrumentation (Fig. 6.13a, b).

6.1.5 Cleaning of the Diamond Crowns

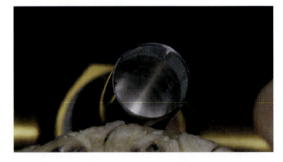

Fig. 6.8 The inner profile of the extractor, combined with a certain roughness, provides consistently safe extraction of the graft

The used diamond instruments are dipped with their crowns in an ultrasonic bath of soapy water (Fig. 6.14a), heated up to a temperature of 60°C and left in the bath for 20 min. After that time, no traces of abrasive wear were detectable on the diamond crown, as was evaluated in the SEM (scanning electron microscope) (Fig. 6.14b). In the case of air-dried instruments which have been used before and which reveal an air-dried coat of bony debris on the diamond crown, the process in the ultrasonic bath should be repeated for another 20 min. The same result can be achieved when used and not yet cleaned, but air-dried instruments are laid in a soapy solution for 30 min and then treated in a normal 20-min process in the ultrasonic bath heated already at a temperature of 60°C.

Fig. 6.9 In removal of the graft cylinder, the extractor remains mounted to the handle and is held upside down in relation to the table, and the bone cylinder is pushed backward out of the tube

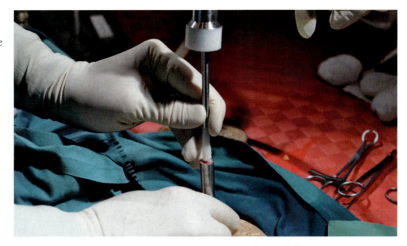

Fig. 6.10 (**a**, **b**) The diamond tool, as well as the extractor, is calibrated along their cylinder mantle

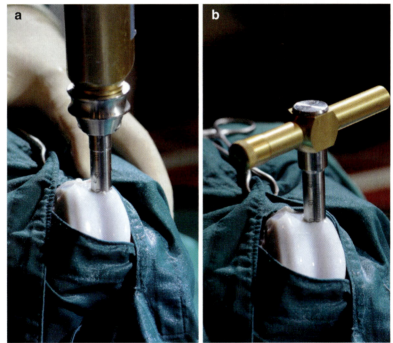

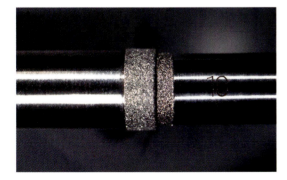

Fig. 6.11 All diamond instruments are designed as twin instruments. The outer diameter of the smaller one is 1/10, 1/15, or even 2/10 mm smaller than the correspondent larger instrument

6.2 Basic Steps of the Operating Technique

6.2.1 Reparation of a Cartilage-Bone Defect

The first step always involves removing the damaged area of the load-bearing joint surface. The size of the removal tube with which the joint surface is first treated, must cut healthy tissue in the transition zone of damaged hyaline cartilage and the healthy remaining surface.

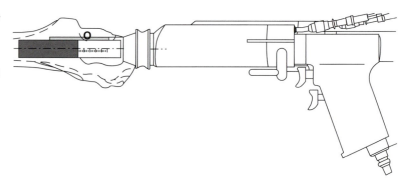

Fig. 6.12 Regarding the inner cooling and rinsing supply, an adapter is available for different suitable drilling machines, providing a cooling line that can be connected to an arthroscopic pump. The diamond instruments are mounted via a quick coupling chuck

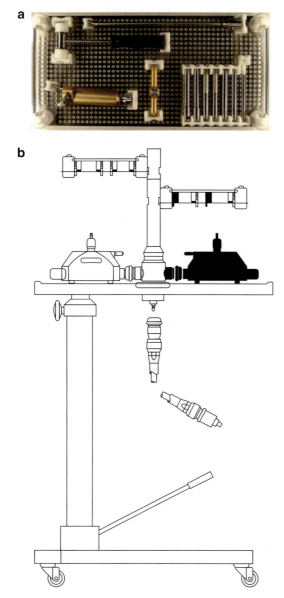

Fig. 6.13 (**a**, **b**) Each set is properly organized within a steritray which can be easily mounted to a modular table for instrumentation

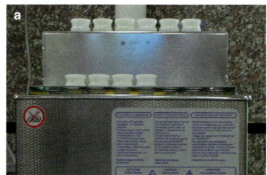

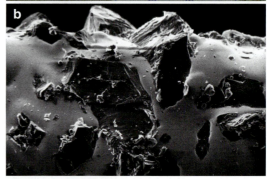

Fig. 6.14 (**a**, **b**) The diamond instrument has to be cleaned in an ultrasound cleaner, heated up to 60°C, and must contain up to 10 ml of liquid soap. After a cleaning period of 20 min, the diamond crown is free of bony debris. In the case of air-dried bone, the process should be repeated for another 20 min

6.2.2 Cutting the Cartilage

The first step in the cartilage-bone transplantation procedure is to sharply cut the cartilage to avoid traumatization by the diamond crown (Fig. 6.15a, b). The diamond hollow grinder is mounted on an adapter fitted with a quick-action chuck. The adapter is attached to a drilling machine equipped with a coolant feedline for the inner lavage visible at the base of the adapter. Once set into the notch that was

6.2 Basic Steps of the Operating Technique

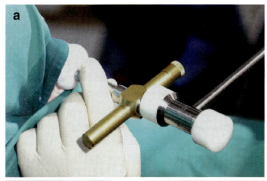

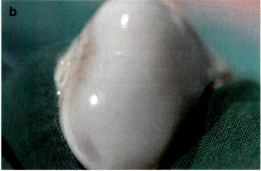

Fig. 6.15 (**a**, **b**) The articular hyaline cartilage, as a soft tissue, should be sharply cut. There is a fine cut visible in the hyaline cartilage. Due to the pattern of the collagenous fibers, the gap opens, and the mineralized bone is accessible for the diamond crown

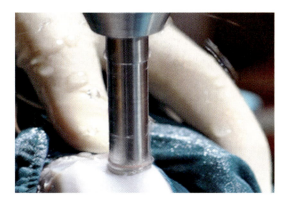

Fig. 6.16 As soon as the compact articular baseplate is ground, the diamond crown should be lifted gently, washing out the debris material

cut by the extractor, the diamond is self-guiding. The nearly constant time of rotation per diameter is about 800–1000 turns per minute. The drill runs at full speed and, after the first 2 mm of penetration,

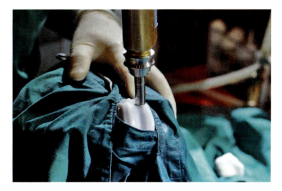

Fig. 6.17 The depth of the penetration of the diamond is defined by the calibration and should be planned preoperatively

the pressure acting on the crown has to be withdrawn until water and debris flows back out of the slot (Fig. 6.16).

Wet-grinding instruments call for more finesse in operation. Internal irrigation to cool the diamond crown and remove swarf can function efficiently only if the pressure on the crown is not excessive and it is occasionally withdrawn a little, care being exercised not to enlarge the hole by this motion. Being a precision operation, grinding calls for more delicacy of touch than the rather cruder process of drilling.

The depth of penetration can be controlled by the calibration on the tube (Fig. 6.17). Once the correct depth has been reached – in a case of osteoarthritis or osteonecrosis, the minimum depth is ensured by reaching the well-vascularized medullary cavity, when blood and especially fat are washed out of the slot – the diamond is removed quickly and at full speed, and the water line is stopped. The fine cut of the thin-walled tool can be visualized (Fig. 6.18); the base of the correctly and artifact-free prepared graft core remains attached to its site. The same-sized extractor – mounted onto the adjustable handle equipped with a quick-action chuck – is now introduced until the depth is reached. This is ensured by the calibrated tool or by the ear because, once the bottom of the slot has been reached, the sound changes distinctly and clearly.

To extract the transplantation core, the removal tube, which has an internal profile (Fig. 6.19a, b), is carefully inserted without any rotational motion. The instrument is gently driven down over the bone core by tapping with the plastic hammer, care being exercised not to hold the device too tightly and thus interrupting the self-guidance of the tool and cutting a "via falsa" with the sharp extractor.

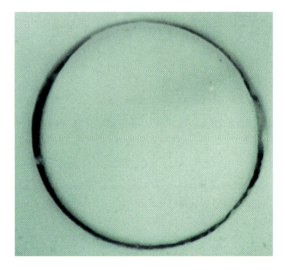

Fig. 6.18 The thin-walled diamond instruments do not remove healthy tissue unnecessarily. The gap for the extractor is very small and should be approached carefully

The graft core is then snapped off in a quick twisting motion (Fig. 6.20a, b).

The extractor, with its handle still mounted, is placed on the instrumentation table upside down and held with two fingers. The core can then be carefully expelled from the tube with a plastic pestle, eccentrically placed on the cut end of the graft core (Fig. 6.21a–c). The cartilage-bone cylinder is preserved in a physiological solution.

The graft is gathered in the same way as described above. The tool with which the transplant is taken out is the corresponding next larger twin. For press-fit fixation, the transplant must be slightly greater in diameter than the recipient site but not so large that implantation conflicts with the cartilage. A carefully validated difference for cartilage-bone cylinders from the epiphysis is worked out and ranges from 1/10–1/20 mm. The validation was focused on the compact cartilage base plate that transfers the load. The bony baseplate should be accurately placed in contact with the recipient cortical wall, similar to a manhole cover that must easily carry the weight of a heavy truck (Fig. 6.22).

Fig. 6.19 (**a, b**) Each graft reveals three little defects which derive from the extractor's inner profile

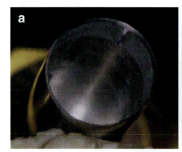
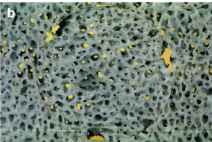

Fig. 6.20 (**a, b**) The extractor is carefully inserted into the gap without any twisting movement, loosely held between thumb and index finger and driven down with gentle blows of the plastic hammer. Once on the ground, the sound changes; with a *quick twisting movement*, the graft is cut off and can be removed with the extractor

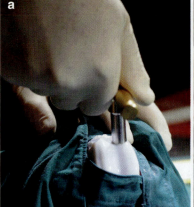
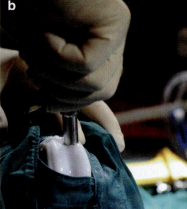

6.2 Basic Steps of the Operating Technique

Fig. 6.21 (**a**) Once in the extractor, the bone graft is removed in a retrograde manner, leaving the extractor mounted to the handle, care being exercised in placing the pusher eccentrically to avoid blowing up the bone graft. (**b, c**) To choose the correct position for the graft, the graft can be placed in the extractor in a retrograde manner. For implantation, it should be placed in an orthograde manner. The cartilage is then pushed into the tube of the extractor which is held upside down

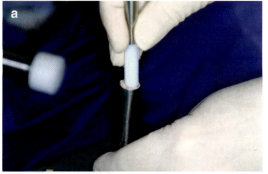
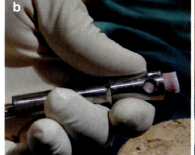
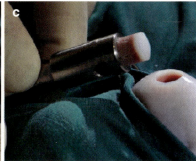

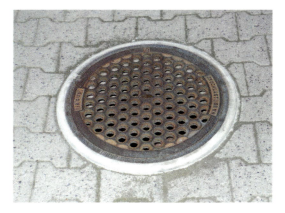

Fig. 6.22 The cylinder is pushed through the extractor until resistance can be felt, then the extractor is carefully removed and, as soon as the cartilage is protected in the recipient defect, the last press-fit of the compact bony baseplate is performed with gentle blows with a hammer on a moist sponge. The graft should fit like a manhole cover, allowing immediate full-load bearing

The length of the graft core should be 1 mm shorter – measured from the bony baseplate – than the depth of the recipient defect. The bony edges of the graft have to be rounded like carpenters' and cabinetmakers' wooden dowels (Fig. 6.23). It is wise to insert some splinters of cancellous bone onto the bottom of the recipient to avoid pushing the graft in too deeply.

Diamond TwInS™ represent the basic principle of a very precise operating technique. All instruments form paired sets: One hollow grinder has an external diameter somewhat smaller than the internal diameter of the next largest instrument which is used to obtain the transplant. The press-fit technique, however, without any screws or wires, calls not only for a very precise instrumental set but also for a skilled surgeon.

The surface contour is carefully compared with the core cylinder of the damaged tissue that was removed, and the prepared graft – the cartilage in front – is then nearly totally inserted into the removal tube without handle in a retrograde manner (Fig. 6.24a, b). The tube protects the hyaline cartilage that only resists compression force. In this way, any shear fracturing of the hyaline tissue can be avoided. For some indications, a special applicator is necessary, i.e., in the ankle joint for talus reconstruction. The removal tube in its new upside-down function is placed with the graft onto the defect. A pestle is inserted into the tube and held rigidly in one hand, whereas the other gently taps on the pestle with a hammer and pushes the graft forward. The graft then passes the window at the end of the tube. The transplant slips into the bed until the baseplate comes up against the rim of compact bone. At this point, the applicator is removed, being careful not to damage

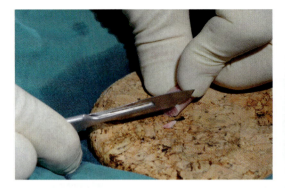

Fig. 6.23 There are some do's and don'ts. As a first step, the edges of the graft should be cut because the cartilage hangs over the defect if the cylinder is removed

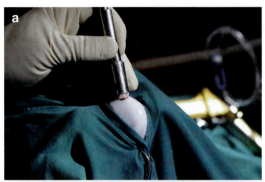

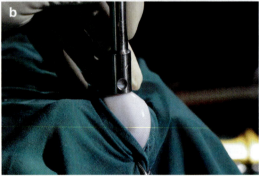

Fig. 6.24 (**a**, **b**) The graft should be carefully placed into the defect because a correction of the position is not possible. The insertion should be controlled through the window of the extractor

the hyaline cartilage by shear stresses. A moist compress is put over the transplant, and a large pestle overlapping the defect is put onto the graft. With gentle blows using a plastic hammer, the graft with its cartilage baseplate is press-fit inserted (Fig. 6.25a). Correctly done, even the hyaline cartilage is press-fit within the remaining healthy tissue (Fig. 6.25b).

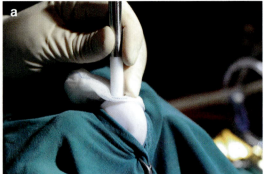

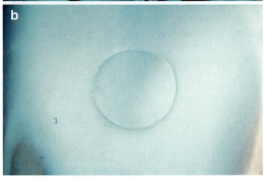

Fig. 6.25 (**a**, **b**) The last gentle blow with a plastic hammer (150 g) should only be performed using a moist compress protecting the hyaline cartilage. The result will be a perfect contact placement of the graft

6.2.3 Reconstructing the Donor Bed

The donor bed for the cartilage-bone graft is, in most cases, the patellar groove, except in the case of femoral head resurfacing. The posterior part of the medial femoral condyle adapts perfectly to the heel-strike area of the femoral head. Due to the upright position of a human being, the hyaline cartilage behind the patella and facing the "coques condyliennes" is subjected to less compressive stress as compared to the flexed position of the knee in most animals (Fig. 6.26a, b). Due to the sliding of the patella, the donor defect has to be reconstructed in a way that the tissue allows sliding of the patella without complaints. Since the cancellous bone in the epiphysis and metaphysis does not heal, the complete defect must be press-fit filled by an osteoconductive ladder of β-TCP. A press-fit β-TCP cylinder is available for each diamond tool, which fills the donor bed perfectly in a way that after resorption,

Fig. 6.26 (**a**) Due to humans' upright position, the patellar groove can act as a donor for healthy hyaline cartilage supported by elastic cancellous bone. (**b**) The function of the femoral condyles has changed as well: In the upright position, the condyles hinder hyperextension. Both areas can serve as donors

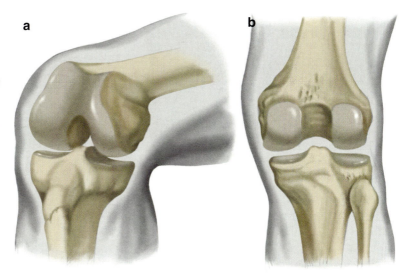

a physiological cancellous bone scaffold is rebuilt (Draenert 2011). Whereas the defect could be reconstructed easily, the reconstruction of the joint surface remained a problem for a long time. Since 2001, the donor bed has been treated with a β-TCP cylinder that has been press-fit inserted. A twin cylinder from the iliac crest providing at least two layers of inserting muscles covers the upper layer of the donor defect up to a depth of 12–14 mm. The cylinder is gathered in a way that the periosteal layer comprising Sharpey's fiber bundles of the abdominal muscles is perfectly preserved (Fig. 6.27a–c). The twin cylinder of the iliac crest presents at its upper pole a roof with a short and steep inclination, and a long and flat one. The roof adapts perfectly to the anatomy of the donor bed. The steep surface is positioned in most cases to the patellar groove, whereas the flat sidepiece faces the outer surface area of the patellar groove. The surface layers of the graft are not as irritable as the hyaline cartilage. For insertion, a pestle can be used in direct contact to the graft. It is of the utmost importance that the bony baseplate of the fiber layers is in contact level with the cartilage baseplate of the donor bed. Since the cartilage is thicker than the fiber layers, the tip of a finger can be dipped into the defect to check the correct placement of the graft (Fig. 6.28).

6.2.4 The Donor Side Morbidity of the Iliac Crest

The round and smooth defects in the iliac crest must be filled in a press-fit manner with a stiff ceramic implant. In all cases, an HA implant is recommended because it must resist the deformation of the iliac crest through the strong abdominal muscles (Fig. 6.29).

6.2.5 Reparation of a Severe Cartilage-Bone Defect

A cartilage trauma or degenerated hyaline surface of more than the width of the defect has to be resurfaced by two or more autologous cartilage-bone grafts. The single procedure is the same. The first step is to remove the damaged tissue. Therefore, the first cylinder that will be taken out is the central cylinder of the weight-bearing area, and the longest graft is replacing the central damaged tissue (Figs. 6.30 and 6.31). The second one overlaps the first, thus providing a sliding runner, and care must be taken not to cut the first graft due to the inclination of the second one: The second one has to be shortened. Since in most cases the first graft protrudes beyond the surface due to the

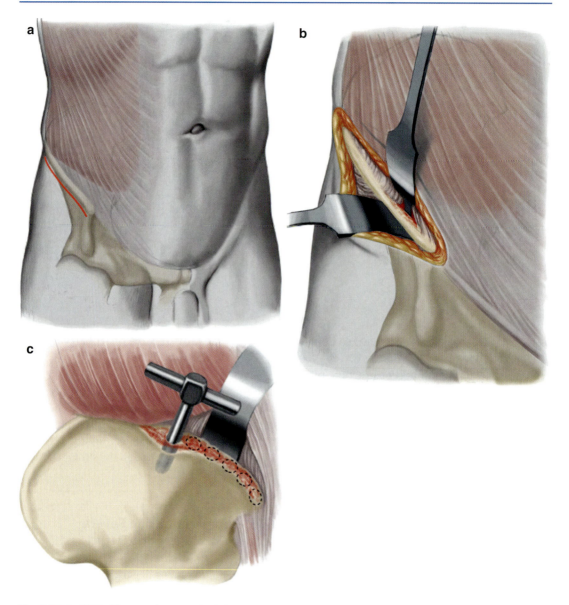

Fig. 6.27 (**a**, **b**) The iliac crest is approached via a slightly laterally placed incision, the subcutis is incised, and the abdominal muscles are preserved and bluntly prepared. One Hohman is placed along the inner wall of the iliac bone, and one is pushed over the lateral balcony of the iliac crest. (**c**) The depth of the graft is limited by the height of the iliac crest. In most cases, the length will not be more than 14–18 mm

thickness of the healthy graft cylinder, the surgeon has to consider the level and inclination of the extractor before cutting the cartilage for the second procedure or to consider an inclined graft. There is a tendency to incline the second graft too steeply (Fig. 6.32); a preoperative planning in a triple graft is therefore necessary (Figs. 6.33 and 6.34).

After the length has been checked carefully, the second cylinder is inserted as described above. As soon as the cartilage baseplate has reached press-fit contact, the applicator tube is removed, and a large pestle is used for the last step of the placement. A moist compress protects the hyaline cartilage, whereas very gentle final blows with the plastic hammer provide a flush seat for the cylinder.

6.2 Basic Steps of the Operating Technique

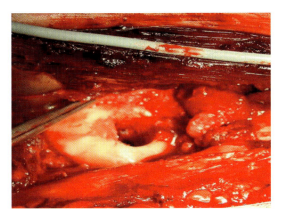

Fig. 6.28 The first step in the reconstruction of the joint's surface is to remove the diseased tissue. The sclerosis defines the depth of the diseased tissue. As soon as the free, fully vascularized cavity is reached, fat marrow and blood appear in the interface, together with the lavage liquid.

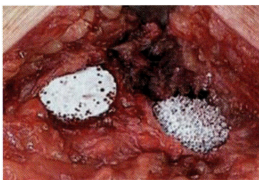

Fig. 6.30 To avoid any donor bed morbidity in the iliac crest, a stiff ceramic implant (Synthacer®) should be press-fit implanted into the defect. The patient should not have any postoperative pain

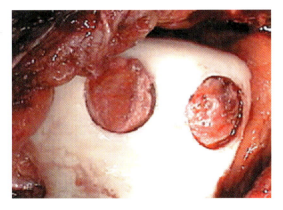

Fig. 6.29 The donor bed has to be refilled completely to avoid preosteoarthritis. Therefore, a press-fit β-TCP implant (Syntricer®) is inserted using the fingers as instrument. Care has to be exercised in inserting the rounded intact cylinder into the donor defect first. After having measured the graft cylinder from the iliac crest, the donor bed with the ceramic is prepared with a sharp spoon until the complete cylinder of the graft can be inserted. The bony baseplate of the graft should be aligned to the cartilage baseplate of the donor bed. The tip of an index finger can be dipped into the defect

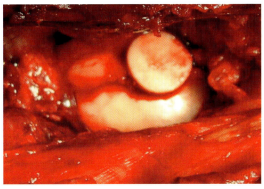

Fig. 6.31 The length of the graft is defined ½ mm shorter than the removed cylinder. The measurement is taken from the tip of the cylinder to the bony baseplate; the cartilage adapts during the following weeks. The bony baseplate, however, does not remodel. Contact healing of the bony baseplate has to be achieved

6.2.6 Reparation of a Complete Condyle with Damaged Cartilage

Very often, the complete condyle has to be reconstructed, and sometimes the level of the joint's surface has already been lost.

The first step of such a reconstruction is again the center of the weight-bearing area. The second and the third cylinders are placed with the necessary inclination and length, care being exercised not to cut the long central cylinder during the placement of the second and third cylinder (Fig. 6.34). The length of the central first graft is defined by the sclerosis, which must be perforated for at least one or two centimeters, thus guaranteeing the revascularization in an osteonecrosis or a remodeling in case of a severe osteoarthritis.

Done well, the contour of the contralateral healthy joint is copied (Fig. 6.35). It might be

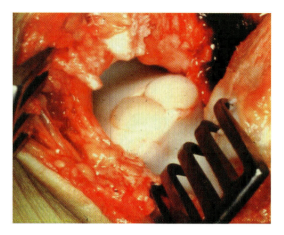

Fig. 6.32 In the case of a double graft, the first cylinder is the longest; the second one has to overlap the main cylinder, providing a sliding runner. The inclination of the second cylinder has to consider the contour of the joint's surface and should be shorter than the first

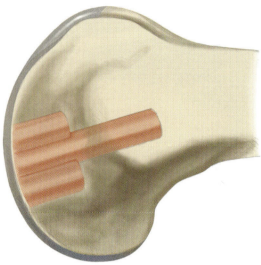

Fig. 6.34 Care has to be exercised not to cut the main central cylinder by a too steeply inclined second or third graft

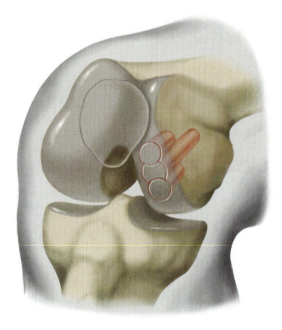

Fig. 6.33 The triple transplant is necessary for reconstruction of a femoral condyle. The first cylinder is the long central one; the accompanying cylinders must be shorter providing a slight inclination. Caution: There is a tendency to create too steep an inclination

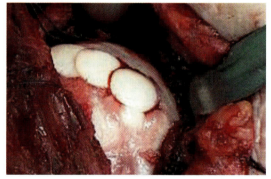

Fig. 6.35 A triple graft has to provide a sliding runner

necessary for the preoperative planning to be performed on the healthy joint mirror image.

The donor defects are furnished with the same combination comprising a press-fit β-TCP cylinder and a twin graft from the anterior half of the iliac crest. The iliac crest itself is provided with HA press-fit cylinders in a way that the patient does not suffer any pain following the operation. Correctly done, there should be no donor bed morbidity at the iliac crest side. As far as the patellar groove is concerned, it takes 3 months until the niveau of the hyaline cartilage is equalized by newly formed fibrocartilage. Rearthroscopies revealed a white bed where it is difficult to define the former donor bed (Fig. 6.36a, b). Immediately after the operation and during passive continuous motion, a rugged sliding is pronounced without complaints and without effusion. The motion will improve as time goes on, and the "noise" will finally disappear after 7–8 weeks.

6.2 Basic Steps of the Operating Technique

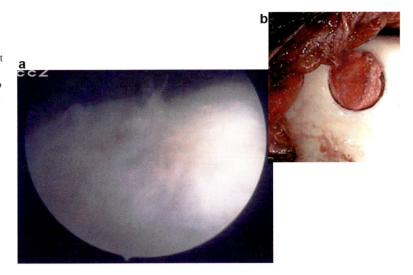

Fig. 6.36 (**a, b**) The reconstruction of the donor bed is of utmost importance: The fiber baseplate should not be placed too high. Dipping the tip of the index finger into the defect guarantees the best control (**b**). Done well, no effusion occurs postoperatively, and the donor bed is refilled with a fibrocartilage within 3–4 months. After 2 years (**a**), it is difficult to find the defect during rearthroscopy

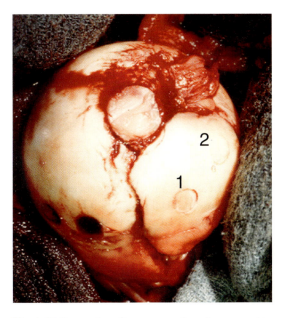

Fig. 6.37 Reparation of an osteocartilage fragment with two cartilage-bone grafts (1 and 2) gathered from the transition zone of the joint. In addition, replacement of the damaged center by a free graft from the lower part of the femoral head

6.2.7 Reparation of an Osteochondral Fragment

The "twin diamond dowelling technique" of osteocartilage fragments represents a procedure where no second intervention is necessary (Fig. 6.37). Compared with all other possibilities, it is the only operation yielding, if well done, a healing ad integrum. The technique described is well known in the area of carpentry and cabinetmaking (Fig. 6.38a, b) and is not entirely new to orthopedic surgery. New is the instrumentation and the standardization and validation of all procedures approached with the precise "twin diamond dowelling technique." The operating technique can be considered as an isoelastic osteosynthesis. Since bone is a living substance, the interface between the interlocking structures will begin to disappear after 1 week and will no longer be visible after 4 weeks. Adaptation to load acting on it will remodel the dowel's structure within the next 20 weeks. This might be different to the carpenters work, but this surgical procedure has its immediate function and biomechanical stability in common with the wooden dowelling technique. The rapidly formed new bone represents the cabinetmaker's glue.

6.2.8 A Tribute to the History of Bone Dowels

Bone chips, struts, and dowels for grafting have been applied more often in orthopedic treatments than in traumatology. Quite obviously, in trauma patients, bone defects have to be treated by filling in with bone chips or substitutes. The biomechanical stabilization, however, is achieved using plates and screws. In orthopedic surgery, stabilization using strong bone chips or struts has been

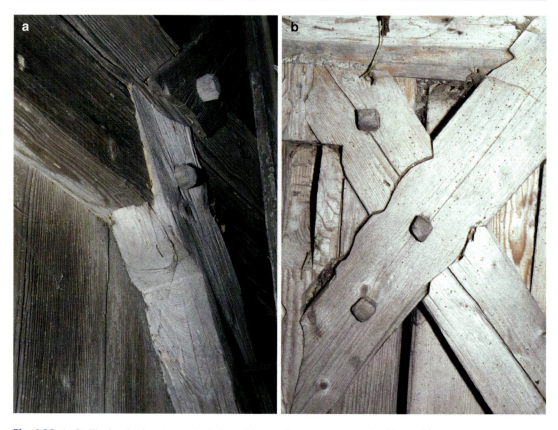

Fig. 6.38 (**a**, **b**) The isoelastic osteosynthesis is well known from carpentry and cabinetmaking

preferred. It seems, however, that during the last 50 years, the metallage with their myriad possibilities for stabilizing fractures have displaced the bone dowelling procedures. This has happened although those procedures were connected with a long list of famous names (Lexer 1908; Lange 1924, 1925; Phemister 1948): individuals who have published an impressive number of excellent and outstanding results. How widespread the bone dowelling techniques once were is documented in textbooks for orthopedic surgeons (Fig. 6.39).

6.2.9 Osteocartilage Fractures

The dowelling technique for osteocartilage fractures using the "twin diamond dowelling technique" represents an operating procedure without rival and is considered the method of choice not only because it avoids a second intervention but also because it is the only known procedure which achieves a restitutio ad integrum (Garde 1995).

The first step is an anatomical reposition using two K-wires for preliminary fixation. The K-wires have to be placed in a perpendicular or slightly divergent position not crossing the course of the planned dowels (Fig. 6.40a–e). Rotational stability is achieved if two dowels can be considered. The first defect is ground in the same way as described for the transplantation. Care has to be taken that the flake has a bony baseplate and is at least 6 mm thick. The cartilage is cut and the underlying bone ground. The lavage system should be carefully controlled because after having passed the fragment, the diamond cooling becomes more difficult, now, that the proximal fragment is in the tube (Fig. 6.40f, g). After having reached the correct depth – at least 12 mm over the fracture gap – the diamond is removed, and the cylinder of the proximal fragment is carefully pushed out of the diamond crown (Fig. 6.41).

6.2 Basic Steps of the Operating Technique

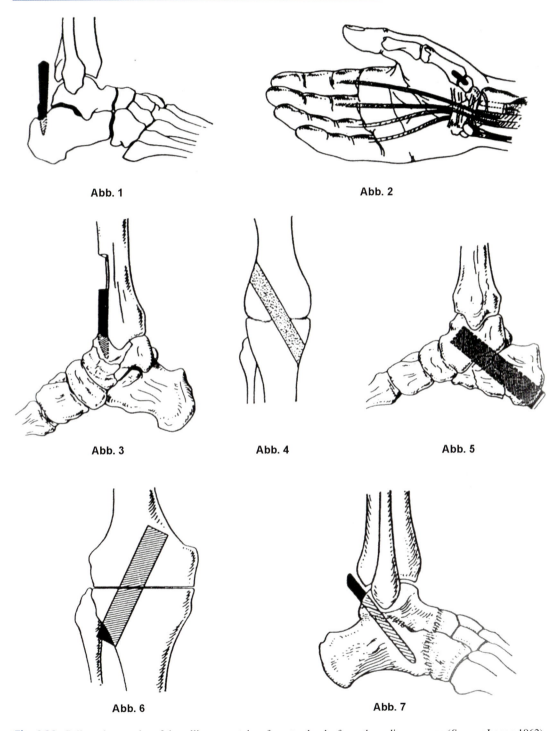

Fig. 6.39 Collected examples of dowelling were taken from textbooks for orthopedic surgeons (*Source*: Lange 1962)

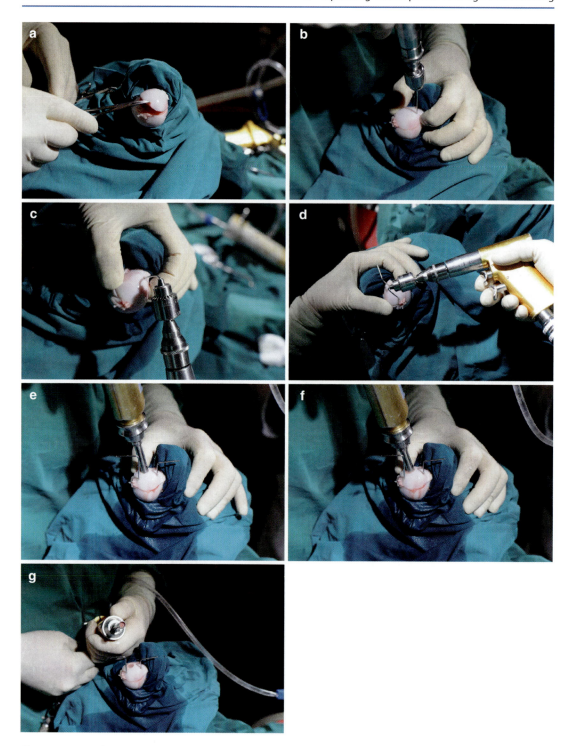

Fig. 6.40 (**a–c**) An osteocartilage fragment has to be refixated preliminarily with K-wires. The path of the wires should not cross the graft dowels. The fragment should have at least 6–8 mm thickness. (**d–f**) Once fixated, the first dowel can be placed, crossing the fracture gap with the small twin diamond. The length of the bed should be not shorter than 10 mm beyond the fracture gap. (**g**) Care has to be applied to remove the fragment cylinder from the diamond tube

6.3 The Donor Bed

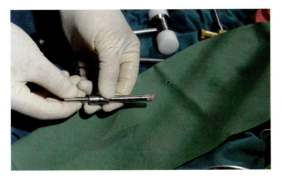

Fig. 6.41 The removal should be done by hand without any hammer

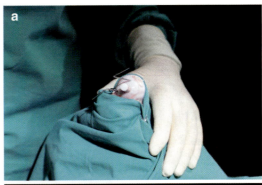

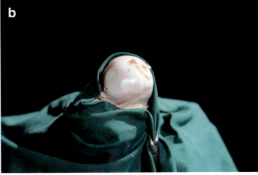

Fig. 6.43 (**a**, **b**) The graft is carefully placed and protected by the extractor. Both grafts are safely in place, and the fragment is stable

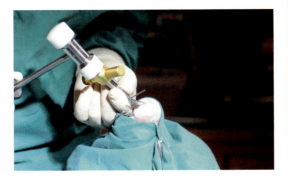

Fig. 6.42 The distal cylinder has to be removed in a second step

The extractor is then placed into the hole and carefully placed over the fracture gap into the slot of the distal fragment (Fig. 6.42). The graft is gathered from the patellar groove or sometimes from the transition zone of the same joint, care being exercised in looking for the best adapted contour of the graft. During insertion of the graft (Fig. 6.43a, b), careful protection of the cartilage is exercised using the extractor "upside down."

The second dowel is placed in the same way reaching an absolute rigid fixation of the osteochondral fragment. In a pig bone with a 10-mm-thick osteochondral fragment, the biological osteosynthesis with two dowels resists a push-out of 5 kg (Fig. 6.44a–c). In case of a fragment or flake, which is too thin, it is safer to remove it and to transplant a new cylinder.

6.3 The Donor Bed

The donor bed is the patellar groove. Due to the upright position of a human being, the cartilage of the patellar groove, as well as the cartilage of the distal femoral condyles adjacent to the coques condyliennes, is exposed to less compressive stress as compared to tetra pods (Fig. 6.45). The donor bed is subdivided into six compartments and, in addition to those areas of the patellar groove (Fig. 6.26a), the lateral condyle and the medial condyle are added as the seventh and eighth donor fields (Fig. 6.26b). If the donor beds are carefully reconstructed, no complaints arise (Figs. 6.46a, b and 6.47a, b).

Up to six cylinders can be gathered from the patellar groove. The area is subdivided in two

Fig. 6.44 (**a–c**) In a pig femoral bone, a refixated segment of the femoral head using two osteocartilage dowels from the patellar groove resist a 5-kg weight hanging on the osteosynthesis

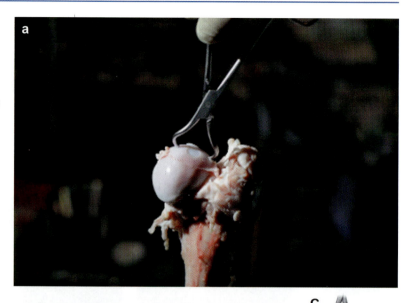
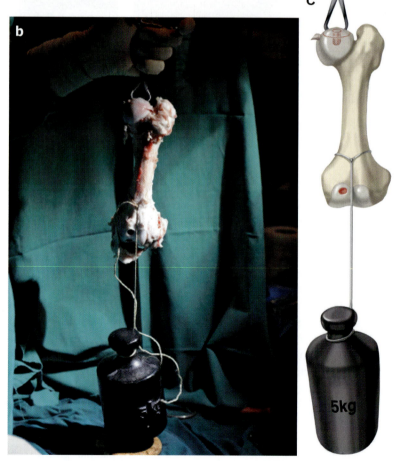

6.3 The Donor Bed

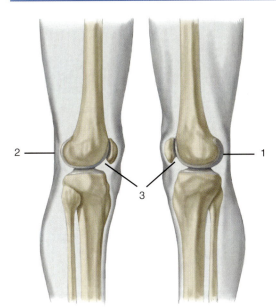

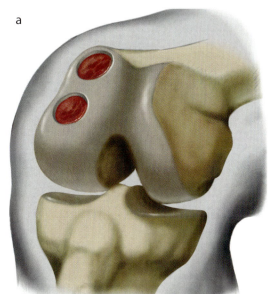

Fig. 6.45 The definition of the donors is important for the success. The stiffer cancellous bone of the posterior condyles (1, 2) and the curvature explain that the medial posterior condyle might be preserved for the femoral and humeral head. The elastic cancellous bone underlying the patellar groove (3) adapts rapidly to the load acting on it in a new recipient bed

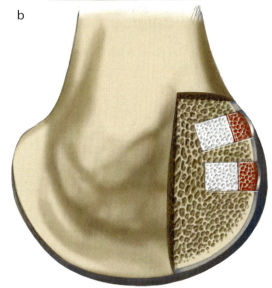

Fig. 6.46 (**a**, **b**) The correct reconstruction of the donor bed comprises the β-TCP press-fit inserted scaffold (Syntricer®) of the whole defect, covered toward the joint by a press-fit cylinder from the iliac crest and providing an intact cambium layer of muscle cells

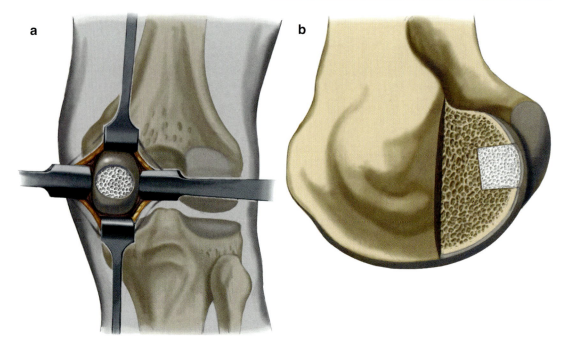

Fig. 6.47 (**a**, **b**) The donor defect of the condyles are reconstructed with a β-TCP cylinder (Syntricer®), press-fit inserted. There is no need for sliding cambium tissue

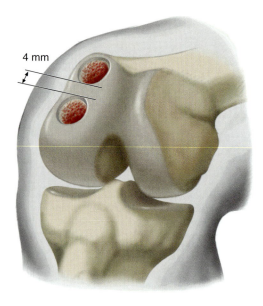

Fig. 6.48 Care has to be exercised to leave an intact bridge of at least 4 mm between two donor defects

lateral segments La_p and La_d (for proximal and distal) and two medial segments Me_p and Me_d; in between are the concave segments Mn_p and Mn_d. Care has to be exercised to preserve at least 4 mm of intact cartilage and bone in between two donor beds (Fig. 6.48).

References

Burkhardt R (1956) Die Myelotomie, eine neue Methode zur kombinierten cytologisch-histologischen Knochenmarksbiospie. Blut 2:267

Draenert K, Draenert Y (1987) Ein neues Verfahren für die Knochenbiopsie und die Knorpel-Knochen-Transplantation. Sandorama III:5–12

Draenert K, Draenert Y, Springorum HW et al (1981) Histo-Morphologie des Spongiosadefektes und die Heilung des autologen Spongiosatransplantates. In: Cotta H, Martini AK (Hrsg) (eds) Implantate und Transplantate in der Plastischen und Wiederherstellungschirurgie. Springer, New York

References

Draenert FG, Mathys R Jr, Ehrenfeld M et al (2007) Histological examination of drill sites in bovine rib bone after in vitro with eight different devices. B J Oral Maxillofac Surg 45:548–552

Draenert K, Draenert M, Erler M et al (2011) How bone forms in large cancellous defects: critical analysis based on experimental work and literature. Injury, Int J Care Injured 42:47–55

Garde U (1995) Histomorphologie der primären Knochenheilung der Osteochondralfraktur. Die knöchernen Umbauvorgänge und restitutio ad integrum im Tierexperiement. Habilitationsschrift Universität, Trnava

Lange F (1924) Die Bolzung der Schenkelhalspseudarthrose. Z Orthop Chir 45:492

Lange M (1925) Entstehung und Behandlung einer Pseudarthrose in einer alten Femurfraktur. Muench med Wschr 72:855

Lange (1962) Orthopädisch-Chirurgische Operationslehre. Zweite Auflage. S.90, 94, 428, 659 and 793. J.F. Bergmann, München

Lexer E (1908) Die Verwendung der freien Knochenplastik nebst Versuchen über Gelenkversteifung und Gelenktransplantation. Langenbecks Arch klin Chir 86:339

Phemister DB (1948) Treatment of pseudarthrosis by simple bone graft without removal of callus. J Int Chir 8:713

Clinical Practice in Autologous Resurfacing®

7.1 Knee

The construction of the knee is an eccentric one. The orientation of the femoral condyles and the tibial plateau favors the flexion of the joint (Fick 1904). Due to the upright position of a human being, the joint's function has changed with the anatomy: The femoral condyles are above, the tibial epiphysis is below, and the patella is in front. The resulting joint does not yet seem fully adapted to this upright position. Under full extension, the knee is in a very stable position protected by the coques condyliennes on the posterior, the collateral ligaments on the medial and lateral side, and the quadriceps muscle including the patella as sesamoid bone anteriorly. As flexion increases allowing rotation of the tibia, the knee becomes more vulnerable and less protected. The histology did not follow the phylogenesis, a fact that can be of use for joint reconstructions. The "facies patellaris" of the patellar groove still reveals a thick hyaline cartilage and an intact elastic underlying cancellous bone in spite of the fact that there is no longer a pronounced and long-lasting pressure acting on it and the stress is more a shear stress by the tangential sliding movement of the patella. The posterior part of the femoral condyle presents mainly cartilaginous protection to avoid hyperextension together with the posterior ligament, the ligamentum posticum Winslowii, or better the "coques condyliennes." Human beings seldom use the hyperflexed position of four-legged animals. The medial condyle reflects the rotational motion on the tibial head and is nicely convex, whereas the lateral condyle looks more like a wheel with different curvatures perpendicular to each other. The posterior part of the femoral condyle can be used as donor, suitable for replacing a damaged heel-strike zone of the femoral head, or in reconstructing a necrotic humeral head.

The approach to the knee joint is a medial one if the medial condyle has to be reconstructed; it is a lateral one if the lateral condyle is concerned (Fig. 7.1a–f).

7.1.1 Trauma

Traumatic osteocartilage defects have a good prognosis if reconstructed at an early stage. Depending on the size of the defect, one (Figs. 7.2a, b and 7.3a–e) or sometimes two press-fit inserted graft cylinders are necessary (Fig. 7.4a–e). A β-TCP cylinder is inserted in the donor bed over the whole length of the defect in the epiphysis and covered toward the joint by a 12–14-mm-thick press-fit cylinder from the iliac crest (Fig. 7.3d). It is important to stabilize the donor defect in the iliac crest with a stiff press-fit ceramic implant. Done well, the patient will not suffer any pain because the deformation of the iliac crest by the strong musculature of the abdominal wall is eliminated.

Seldom does trauma lead to large cartilage decollement, i.e., if long-lasting overloading has taken place as might happen during excessive dancing as shown in the young student (Fig. 7.5a).

78   7 Clinical Practice in Autologous Resurfacing

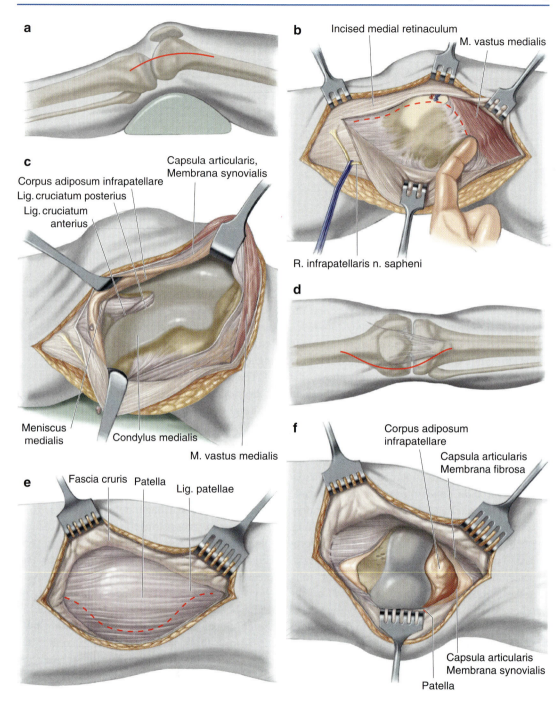

Fig. 7.1 (**a–f**) The medial approach is done in a parapatellar manner. The retinaculum has to be incised such that it is closed to the patella in order to avoid cutting the medial vaste of the quadriceps muscle, the incision should follow the tendon close to the patella. The lateral incision is performed in the same way. The Hohman's hooks can be placed along the basis on the lateral or medial metaphyseal wall and over the tip of the patella into the notch

7.1 Knee

Fig. 7.2 (**a, b**) A single traumatic lesion will be reconstructed with one graft carefully chosen with respect to the surface contour (Garde, Iserlohn)

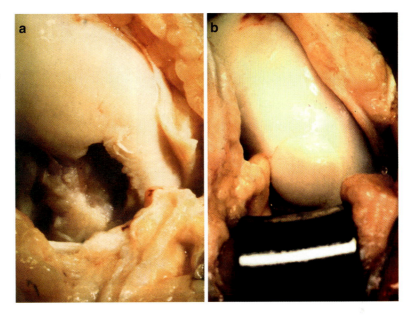

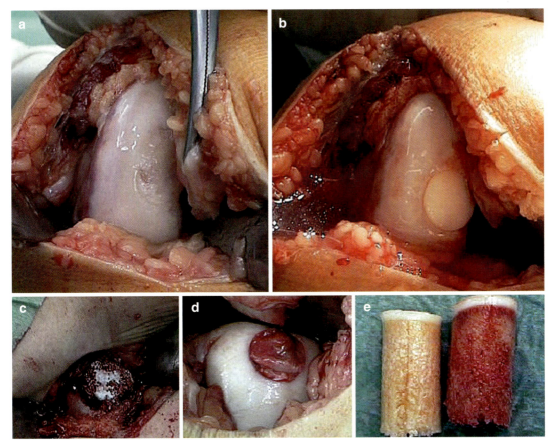

Fig. 7.3 (**a–e**) The diseased tissue has to be removed completely, and the graft should contact healthy cartilage. The donor bed in the iliac crest is to be refilled immediately with a stiff ceramic in a press-fit manner, the donor bed carefully reconstructed providing a cambium layer. In most cases, vascularization is impressively different in the donor graft

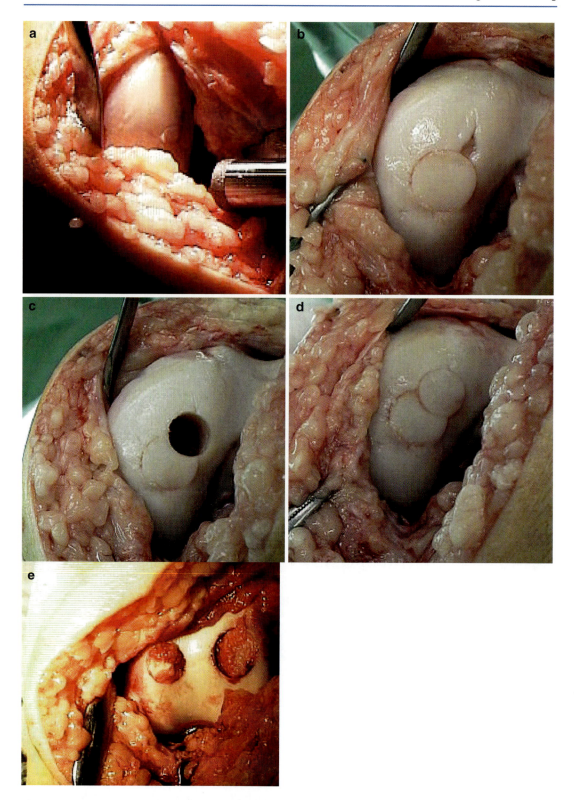

Fig. 7.4 (**a–e**) A double grafting procedure has to be taken into consideration as a sliding runner. The first and main graft is the long one; the second should be slightly inclined and shorter

7.1 Knee

It is necessary to reconstruct a thorough-going surface where the grafts interlace, resulting in load-bearing support without any gaps (Fig. 7.5b).

7.1.2 Osteochondritis Dissecans

As soon as the "quiet necrosis" (Paget 1870), the "osteochondritis dissecans" of König (1888), has yielded a loose body, the removal of which was first described by Ambroise Paré (1841), the reconstruction is probably the only possibility to yield a restitutio ad integrum. As long as no dissection is observed, any conservative treatment focusing on non-weight-bearing might be successful, especially in young children (Green and Banks 1990). Internal fixation (Adachi et al. 2009) and mosaicplasty (Bentley et al. 2003) did not fulfill the expectations. The etiology of the disease is multifactorial and inhomogeneous (Gardiner 1955; Aichroth 1971; Bruns 1996; Yonetani et al. 2010).

In young patients, the anatomical reconstruction is important. Sometimes, a template taken from the contralateral healthy joint has to be prepared, i.e., to elevate the load-bearing surface of the "stand phase" of the knee's medial condyle (Fig. 7.6a–g). Care has been exercised in order that the bony cartilage baseplate of the new plateau can heal in contact and all grafts are interlaced (Fig. 7.6e, g). The same care has to be applied to the reconstruction of the donor defects: The bony anchoring plate of Sharpey's fiber bundles of the abdominal muscles should be aligned with the cartilage baseplate. The tip of the indicator finger will fit into the defect. The iliac crest graft is press-fit inserted, and there is no effusion caused by the donor defects if carefully done (Fig. 7.6f).

Sometimes, the necrosis overlaps the edge of the notch, thus yielding partly unconstrained grafts after reconstruction (Fig. 7.7a–e). A non-weight-bearing period of 4 weeks is considered adequate for the contact healing of the cancellous bone. In young individuals, a restitutio ad integrum can be expected.

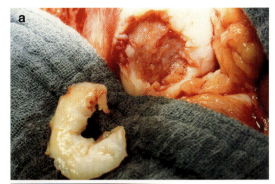
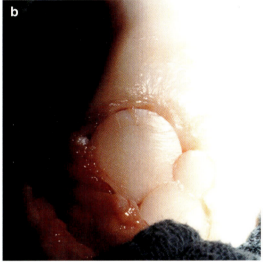

Fig. 7.5 (**a**, **b**) A traumatic décollement can occur. In this example, a young dancer has fatigue-loaded the joint, resulting in a huge décollement. A triple transplant was necessary to cover the defect (Garde, Iserlohn)

7.1.3 Osteoarthritis

In osteoarthritis, the degenerative joint disease usually passes a phase of synovial inflammation. As far as the etiology is concerned, the inhomogeneous group reveals in all stages fissures, defects or craquelé fractures, or smaller or larger defects of the hyaline cartilage. In all affected joints, the underlying bone is severely altered, revealing sclerosis and deformation including the formation of osteophytes. The reconstruction of those articular joint surfaces, as far as no rheumatoid inflammation is concerned, is successful if the diseased tissue of the

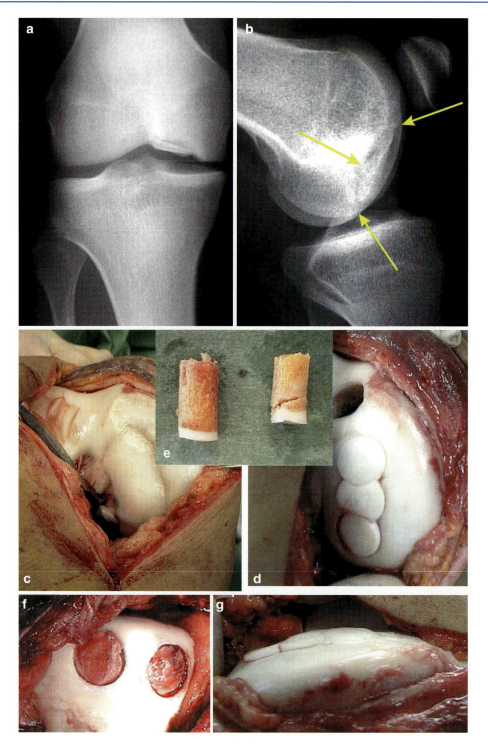

Fig. 7.6 (**a–g**) Osteochondritis dissecans involves young active individuals, very often high-level athletes. An 18-year-old soccer player was reconstructed relifting the joint plateau. Ten years later, the young man is a motocross rider

7.1 Knee 83

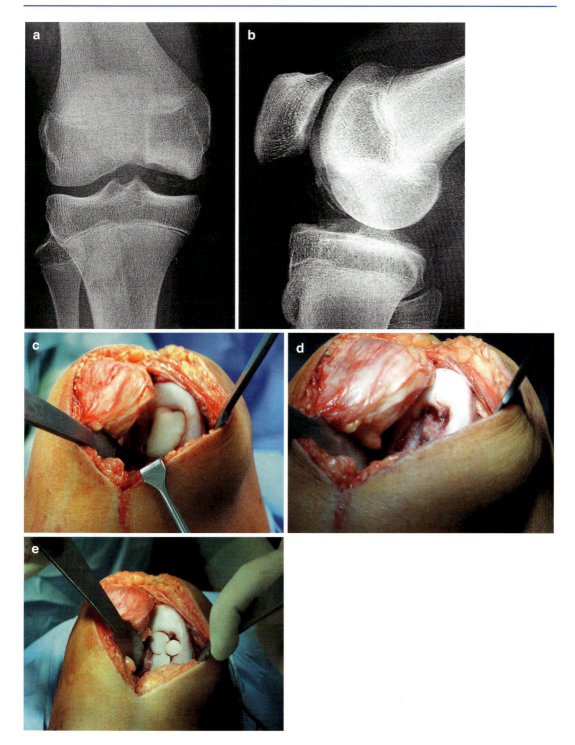

Fig. 7.7 (**a–e**) In this 14-year-old female patient, the segment was already loose and thus replaced with three long osteocartilage grafts from the patellar groove. The follow-up is now 4 1/2 years

epiphysis is removed and the load-transferring cartilage baseplate is nicely reconstructed. The sclerosis has to be totally removed and replaced by intact and elastic cancellous bone, which in most cases is still available in the patellar groove. Careful reconstruction is rewarded with long-lasting results (Fig. 7.8a–c). The 50-year-old female was operated on 14 years ago. Three years after operation, a rearthroscopy revealed an intact and fully recovered hyaline joint surface. The woman still enjoys full motion without an artificial joint.

It is surprising what results can be achieved if the operation is carefully performed, the new load-transferring baseplate can heal in contact, if all osteophytes are removed and also if the counter partner in the tibial head is replaced by healthy tissue (Fig. 7.9a–i). In severe osteoarthritis, joint reconstructions have been performed in patients who refused to have their joint replaced. In this 74-year-old woman, the state several years after a varisation osteotomy (a, b) had yielded bone-to-bone articulation (c). The osteophytes were removed, 25° of the condylar load-bearing area was resurfaced, and the niveau lifted 4 mm, allowing the baseplate of the cartilage (d) to heal in contact. The grafts from the patella groove revealed elastic spongious bone and intact hyaline cartilage, and the tissue taken out was malvascularized and brittle (e). In the tibial head, a periosteal bone graft was press-fit inserted, and all three donor beds in the patellar groove were carefully filled with press-fit cylinders from the iliac crest including two layers of the abdominal muscles. The niveau of the fiber baseplate was en niveau with the cartilage baseplate. Care was taken such that the reconstructed condyle allowed a smooth gliding movement on the tibial plateau without any interlocking. CPM (continuous passive motion) was applied postoperatively. Load bearing was allowed starting with 12 kg, slowly increasing to full weight after 6 weeks. All donor defects in the iliac crest were filled in a press-fit manner with a hydroxyapatite (Synthacer®) cylinder (Fig. 7.9h). The patient did not suffer pain and there was no iliac crest morbidity and no hematoma.

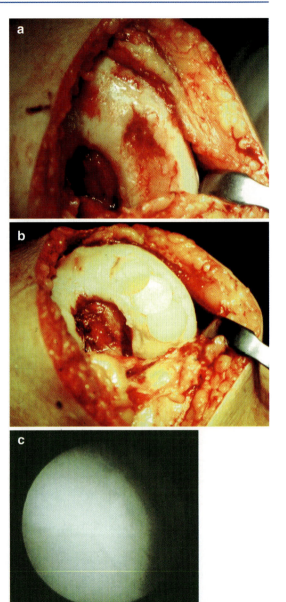

Fig. 7.8 (a–c) The complete destruction of the articular surface was nicely reconstructed 14 years ago. Three years after the operation, the patient underwent a rearthroscopy which revealed complete recovery of the sliding runner of the condyle. The patient is still free of complaints and fully active (Rischke, Hamburg)

Craquelé fractures of the hyaline cartilage are very common in high-level athletes, as shown here in a "gold medal winner." In most cases, jumping athletes demonstrate severe sclerosis of the underlying cancellous bone, which has to be removed up to a depth of 35–40 mm (Fig. 7.10a, b).

7.1 Knee

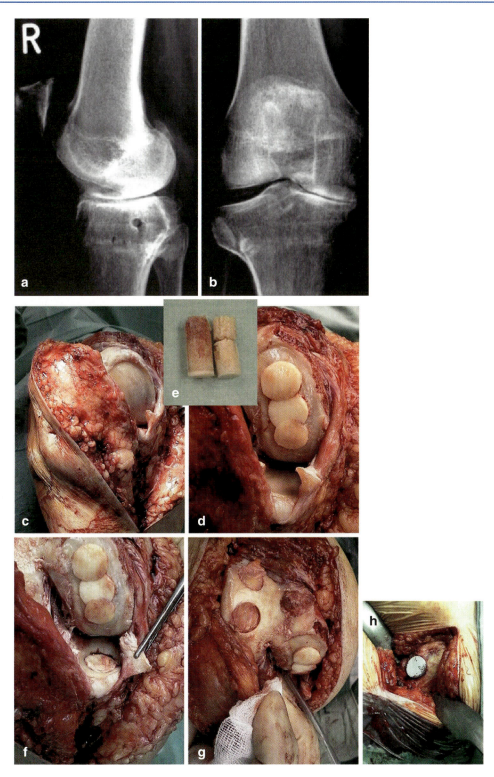

Fig. 7.9 (**a–i**) The 74-year-old patient had an osteotomy several years ago and rejected joint replacement. The reconstruction considered a sliding runner of the medial condyle, removal of all osteophytes, and proper reconstruction of the donor beds. The tibial head was medially reconstructed with a cylinder covered with periosteum. The woman left the hospital 10 days after surgery and, 10 years later, is still an active biker without an artificial joint

Fig. 7.9 (continued)

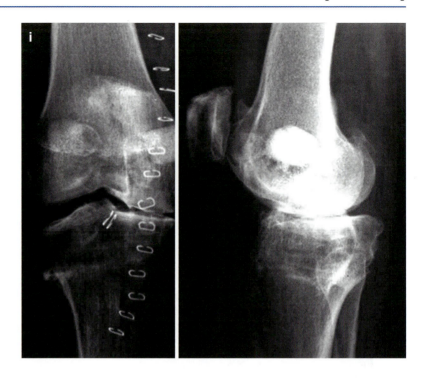

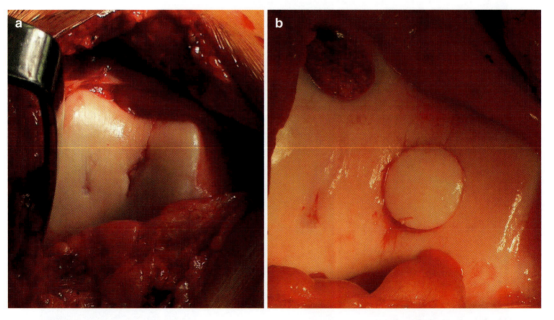

Fig. 7.10 (**a**, **b**) A high-level volleyball player (gold medal winner) suffered severe pain during jumping. The 1-cm-deep sclerosis in the patellar groove was removed and replaced by a healthy graft. The athlete recovered quickly and is playing again (2-year follow-up) (Thomas, Los Angeles)

7.2 Ankle Joint and Foot

7.2.1 Trauma

In August 2001, one of the authors operated on a severe osteoarthritis of the ankle comprising a destroyed tibial, as well as a destroyed talus joint surface (Fig. 7.11a–c). It was the first time that the talus dome had been reconstructed through the distal tibial bone. The Diamond TwInS™ technology was used (Fig. 7.11d–i). The instrument sets comprise an uninterrupted series of tools (§9 ff). Using a diamond tool two sizes larger (16.3 mm) than the tools used for grafting the talus, the tibia was cut approaching the talus dome. The talus dome was reconstructed with two 12.85-mm measuring grafts. As a last step, the concave tibial joint surface was replaced in a retrograde manner with a press-fit graft measuring 16.45 mm. All three grafts were gathered from the patellar groove. In spite of the press-fit seat, a transverse K-wire was necessary to avoid displacement of the graft during deformation of the epiphysis under load (Fig. 7.11h). All cartilage donor beds were carefully press-fit stabilized with grafts comprising bone and a cambium layer of muscle cells and periosteum, respectively. Donor defects larger than 15.25 mm (TL 13) have to be filled with periosteum-bone grafts gathered from the distal medial femoral condyle. Care has to be exercised not to remove the adhering periosteum. They were taken from the iliac crest and the medial metaphysis of the femur; all bone defects were press-fit filled by a fully interconnected HA implant (Synthacer®*), thus avoiding deformation and donor bed morbidity (Fig. 7.11g, i). The patient left the hospital on the sixth day postoperatively and started weight bearing after 6 weeks. The control after 2 years showed full function and a 100% Lyshom's score (Fig. 7.11e, j).

A 20-year-old woman suffering a pilon fracture on her left ankle joint was operated on in an emergency situation, leaving a large defect in the tibial joint plateau and, as a result, a talus tilt fixed by the adjusting screw (Fig. 7.12a). Two weeks after the emergency operation, the revision was preplanned (Fig. 7.12b). During the operation, the medial plate was removed, as was the adjusting screw. The fibula osteosynthesis, however, was left intact. Using Diamond TwInS™ technology, the defect in the distal tibial plateau was approached transosseously and a 15.25-mm graft from the patellar groove was press-fit inserted in a retrograde manner. The medial malleolous was displaced 3 mm distally and the plate refixated in the new position. The graft was fixated by a transverse K-wire as described above (Fig. 7.12c). Six weeks after the operation, the K-wire was removed and weight bearing started with 12 kg and full weight after 8 weeks. The control after 12 weeks revealed nice reconstruction of the tibia and a talus in correct position (Fig. 7.12d).

7.2.2 Osteochondritis Dissecans (Talus)

Quite obviously, a familiar disposition is prevalent as far as the osteonecrosis of the talus is concerned. We report on 18-year-old twin girls who were active top league volleyball players suffering identical dome necrosis of the right talus. Both were operated on in June 2001. The medial approach is marked by a steep osteotomy of the medial malleolus starting at the medial edge of the talus in a sagittal direction, thus giving way to a perpendicular approach to the talus' joint surface, which appears multifractured and loose (Fig. 7.13a–e). Both girls showed the same lesion (Fig. 7.14a, b). Cartilage and baseplate had been already dissected (Fig. 7.14c, d). A 14.05-mm (TL12) graft was press-fit inserted in a 13.90-mm defect (Fig. 7.14e). The nicely convex graft was gathered from the medial condyle of the patellar groove (Fig. 7.14f). The graft formed the edge of the talus and was unconstrained in the upper fourth. Weight bearing therefore did not start before the sixth week. The donor bed was filled with a β-TCP ceramic and a press-fit cylinder from the iliac crest, providing a cambium layer with pluripotential mesenchymal cells (Fig. 7.14g). Finally, the iliac crest donor bed was

Fig. 7.11 (**a–j**) The first transosseous reconstruction of the ankle joint was performed in 2001. The tibial tunnel measured 16.3 mm. The talus dome was reconstructed with two grafts measuring 12.85 mm. The control was done with the arthroscope (**e**). The tibial surface was covered in a retrograde manner with a graft measuring 16.45 mm, the donor bed of which was reconstructed with a periosteal covered metaphyseal graft (**h**). The patient demonstrated full function 2 years postoperatively (**i, j**)

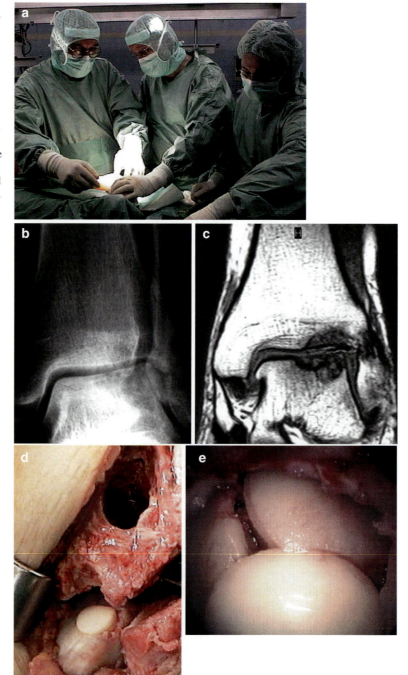

7.2 Ankle Joint and Foot

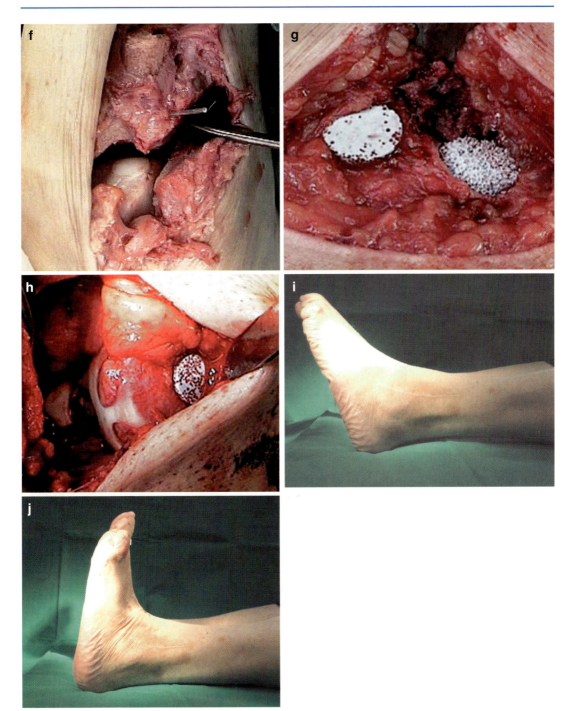

Fig. 7.11 (continued)

Fig. 7.12 (**a–d**) Preoperative planning of the revision of a pilon tibial in a 20-year-old woman was the basis for the reoperation. Five-year result

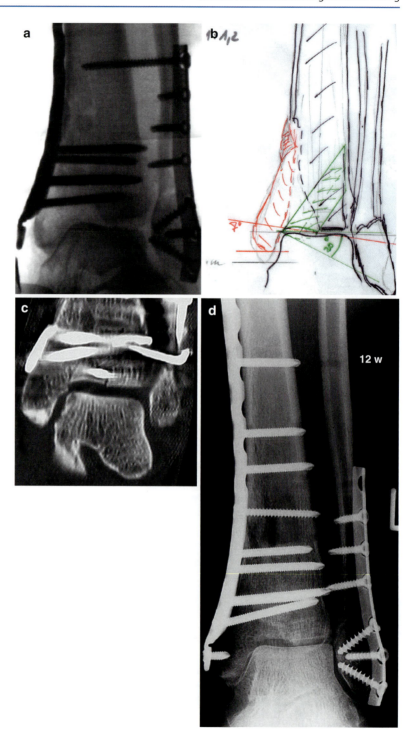

7.2 Ankle Joint and Foot

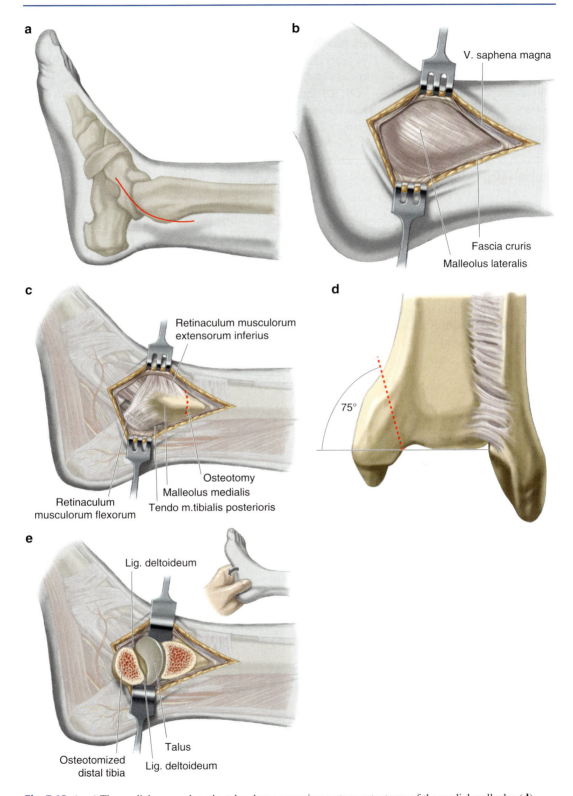

Fig. 7.13 (a–e) The medial approach to the talus dome comprises a steep osteotomy of the medial malleolus (d)

stabilized by a fully interconnected HA implant (Fig. 7.14h). The osteotomy had been stabilized with two cancellous bone screws. Five years after the operation, function and NMR showed a restitutio ad integrum in both girls (Fig. 7.14i, j). Even more pronounced was a deep necrosis of the talus in a 16-year-old girl, treated in December 2001 with a 10.60-mm graft (Fig. 7.15a–d). The lateral approach is performed with a steep osteotomy of the fibula (Fig. 7.16a–e).

7.3 Hip and Pelvis

The approach to the hip joint with surgical dislocation is advantageously performed using the Kocher-Langenbeck incision and the flip osteotomy described by Ganz et al. (2001) and based on anatomical studies focused on the medial circumflex artery (Gautier et al. 2000) (Fig. 7.17a–e).

7.3.1 Trauma

Osteosyntheses of the pelvis sometimes neglect the acetabulum. In most cases, the consequences are severe with respect to the hip joint. A 27-year-old man was externally treated with an osteosynthesis (Fig. 7.18a); however, he suffered severe pain during motion of the left femur. The CT scan revealed the penetration of one screw tangentially into the hip joint (Fig. 7.18b). The revision operation presented a décollement of the hyaline cartilage of the complete stand phase and part of the toe-off phase (Fig. 7.18c). The heel-strike phase was still intact. The hyaline cartilage of the stand phase was reconstructed using the Diamond TwInS™ technology (Fig. 7.18d). The cartilage of the toe-off phase was not replaced. After 12 weeks, the CT scan revealed nice reconstruction of the femoral head (Fig. 7.18e, f). The patient was reintegrated into his job and did well without any restriction for 2½ years. After that time, pain reoccurred during a short walk, and he was operated on again for a hip replacement. The operating situs revealed a persistent defect in the acetabulum where the screw had entered the joint. A large cyst had developed in the roof of the acetabulum and was quite obviously responsible for the complaints. The autologous grafts inserted in the stand phase of the head were well integrated and revealed healthy hyaline cartilage.

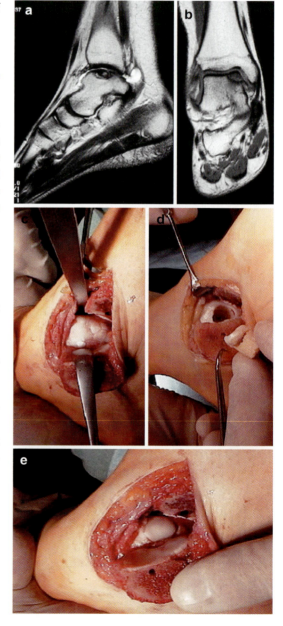

Fig. 7.14 (**a–h**) Twin high-level athletes suffering osteochondritis dissecans. Both 18-year-old girls were active volleyball players. They were operated in 2001. Both patients healed ad integrum (**i, j**)

7.3 Hip and Pelvis

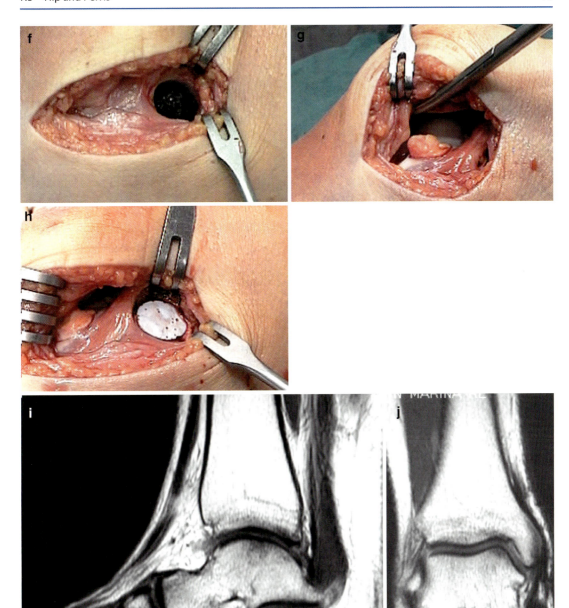

Fig. 7.14 (continued)

In a 20-year-old male, a pelvis fracture was stabilized by an osteosynthesis, leaving a gap open in the roof of the acetabulum. The patient was considered for an internal acetabuloplasty, which was performed in the September 2008 the first time (Fig. 7.19a). The former spheroid acetabulum revealed a more ellipsoid one, and a screwed femoral head like a protrusion of the acetabulum (Fig. 7.19b, c). The rotation of the joint was completely blocked. After preoperative

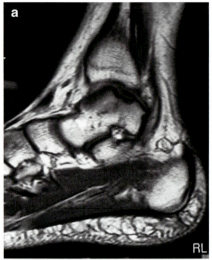

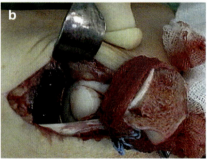

Fig. 7.15 (a–d) A complete necrosis of the talus dome in a 16-year-old girl was treated with a partly unconstrained graft. There was nonload bearing prescribed for 6 weeks, resulting in perfect function with restitutio ad integrum

planning for a new medial support in the acetabulum, the revision was performed on the open joint via a posterolateral approach according to Kocher-Langenbeck, and a flip osteotomy (Ganz et al. 2001). The gap in the acetabulum was prepared and a new medial support was formed using three autologous cartilage-bone grafts from the patellar groove. A posterior approach behind the femoral neck was thus used to reach the acetabulum perpendicular to its surface (Fig. 7.19d, e). The already damaged femoral head was reconstructed with a fourth large graft from the patellar groove (Fig. 7.19f). Immediately after reposition of the femoral head, its internal rotation was free again. The patient left the hospital 10 days after the operation and was allowed weight bearing after 16 weeks. He is back in his job and the joint has been doing well for 3 years.

7.3.2 Heel-Strike Osteoarthritis

Evaluation of the locomotion forms the basis in defining loads acting on circumscribed articular surface areas. The mechanics of locomotion were first investigated by the Weber brothers (1836); the more precise mathematical calculation along rigid mathematical lines was performed by Otto Fischer (1903). Fischer made his calculations with the support of the King of Saxon: With the help of the 8th Royal Saxonian Infantry of Prince Johann Georg Nr. 107, Fischer collected all data on the normal human gait which then enabled him to identify 41 phases of the gait (Fig. 7.20). His calculated diagraphs were close to the kinematical analysis und presentation of Marey (1884) (Fig. 7.21). Gait analysis starts with the "toe-off" phase (0) and ends with the "heel-strike" phase (41); in between, we identify the foot-to-ground phase (16–24). During the heel-strike phase, the anterior third of the femoral head is loaded. Depending on the dynamics of the gait, the load acting on the anterior part of the femoral head is measured up to 4.5 times body weight (Pauwels 1935), whereas in the toe-off phase, less than 15% of the weight is loaded on to the posterior third of the articular surface of the femoral head (Diehl 1976).

In osteoarthritic hips, the heel-strike phase of the femoral head presents in most subjects the most pronounced abrasion (Fig. 7.22), whereas the rest of the head shows a physiological hyaline cartilage.

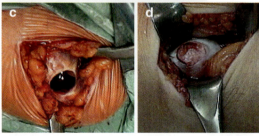

Fig. 7.16 (a–e) The lateral approach to the talus dome comprises a steep osteotomy of the fibula and the tubercle of Tillaux-Chaput (d)

7.3 Hip and Pelvis

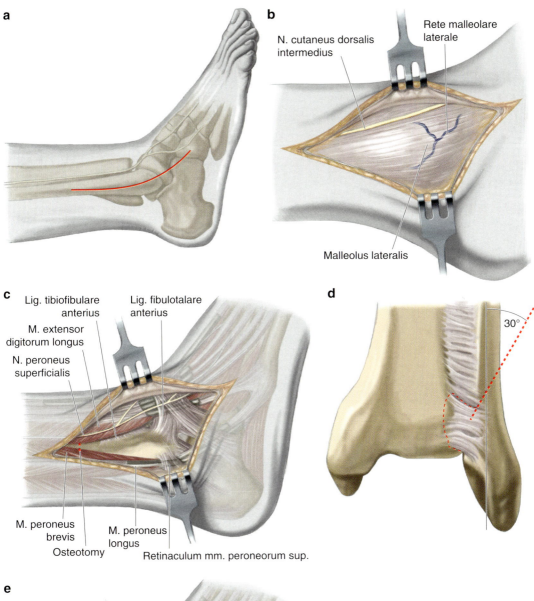

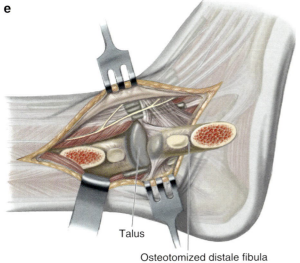

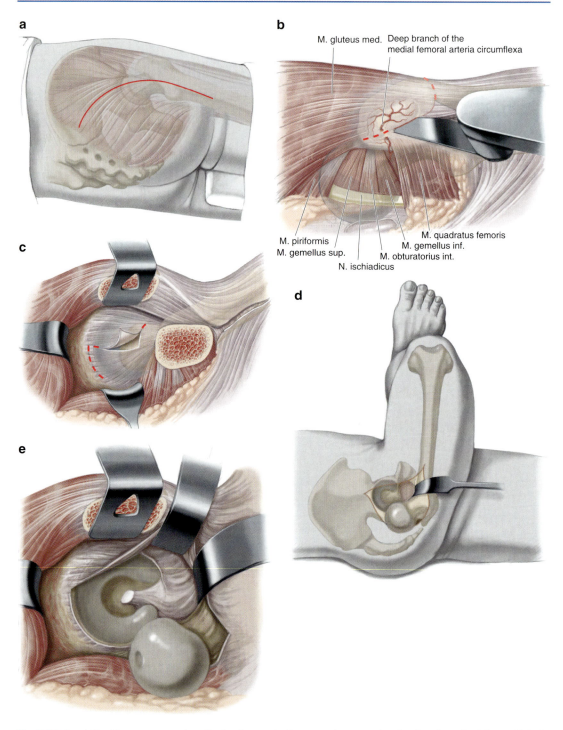

Fig. 7.17 (a–e) The flip osteotomy via a Kocher-Langenbeck approach, preserving the deep branch of the medial circumflex artery

7.3 Hip and Pelvis

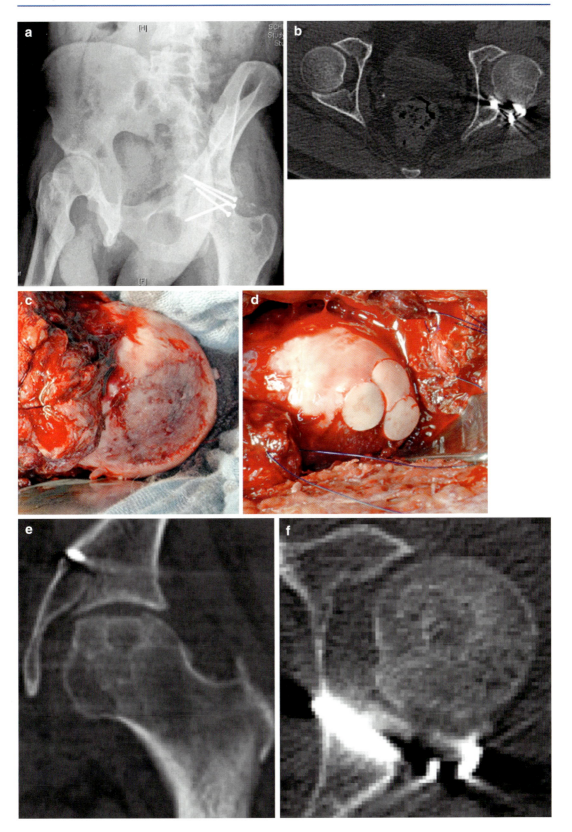

Fig. 7.18 (**a–f**) Décollement of the femoral head and reconstruction of the area of the stand phase. The 27-year-old patient was outside operated on. The revision was performed at the University of Homburg

Fig. 7.19 (**a–f**) Revision of a pelvis fracture leaving a gap in the acetabulum and yielding protrusion of the femoral head with its destruction. A reconstruction of a new medial wall was performed with perfect results following the intervention. Three-year follow-up

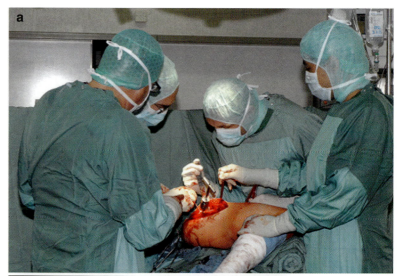

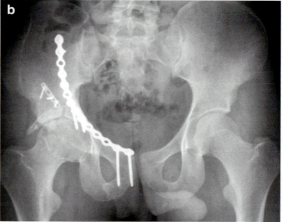

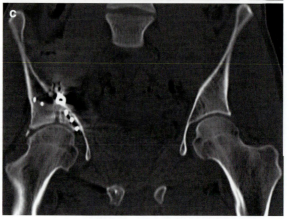

Fig. 7.19 (continued)

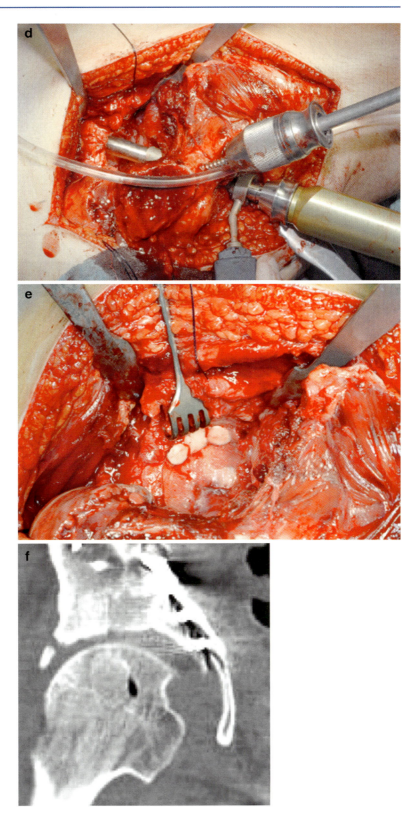

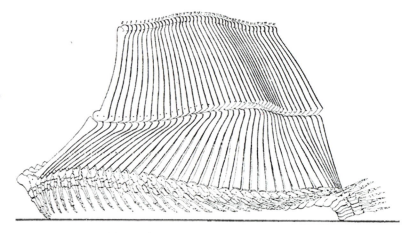

Fig. 7.20 The 41 phases of the human gait were calculated by Otto Fischer and comprise the initial "toe-off" (0) and the final "heel-strike" phase (41) (*Source*: Fischer 1903, Fig. 8)

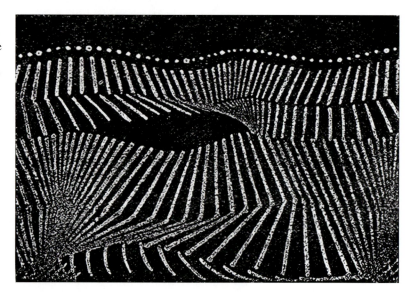

Fig. 7.21 Marey's kinematical analysis of the human gait was published 19 years before Fischer's exact calculation (*Source*: Fischer 1903, Fig. 1)

The anterior part of the femoral head can be approached by a direct medial incision without dislocation of the femoral head. After opening of the capsule by means of a "Z"-incision, the anterior part of the femoral head is exposed in hyperextension, and the articular surface can be reconstructed with three grafts from the ipsilateral knee, advantageously, a large graft from the posterior distal medial femoral condyle is used (Fig. 7.23a–f). In a patient, a 42-year-old man, via a medial approach, the heel-strike phase was exposed, and the necrotic tissue was removed and replaced with a triple graft (Fig. 7.24a–d). The man left the hospital on the fifth day, loaded the joint physiologically beginning after the 12th week, and was free of complaints at a follow-up after 4 years (Fig. 7.24e).

7.4 Shoulder

The main indication in a shoulder joint is a lesion following dislocation of the humerus, which might be a typical or a sometimes atypical "Hill-Sachs" lesion, revealing an impressive fracture of

7.6 Hand and Wrist

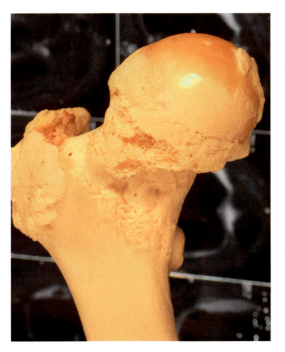

Fig. 7.22 Heel-strike osteoarthritis due to loading of the anterior third of the femoral head in a heel-strike phase which exceeds 4.5 times body weight. The blanc's bone contrasts the intact cartilage layer with the rest of the femoral head

the humeral epiphysis. In most cases, the lesion is responsible for recurrent dislocations.

The anterior approach through the subscapularis muscle and the articular capsule presented the deep impression in the humeral head of the 21-year-old man suffering recurrent dislocations of his right shoulder (Fig. 7.25a–c). The impression was treated with three osteochondral grafts taken from the patellar groove. The patient has been free of a recurrence since that operative intervention.

A 31-year-old male patient suffered an osteonecrosis of the left humeral head, yielding a completely lost contour in the center of the convex articular surface (Fig. 7.26a–c). Due to the equally convex contour, the graft was gathered from the medial condyle of the distal femur (Fig. 7.26d). The 35-mm-long graft exactly reconstructed the humeral articular surface (Fig. 7.26e). The patient is still free of complaints 17 months following the operation.

7.5 Elbow

In a 42-year-old truck driver, osteoarthritis had destroyed the humero-radial joint. The articular surfaces were approached transosseously under control of the endoscope using the Diamond TwInS™ technology (Fig. 7.27a–c). The articular surface of the caput radii was replaced through the osseous tunnel in the condylus radialis humeri, yielding a perfect reconstruction of the foveal surface. The articular surface of the humeral condyle was transplanted in a retrograde manner and fixated by a K-wire for 6 weeks. The X-ray revealed precise reconstruction; osteophytes were not removed anteriorly. Twelve weeks following the operation, the patient was back in his job, and 4 years later, he was still free of complaints (Fig. 7.27d–f).

7.6 Hand and Wrist

A comminuted fracture of the distal radius in a 42-year-old woman was treated using screw and K-wire osteosynthesis as well as a disk transplant from the iliac bone using the diamond instruments. The disk could be press-fit inserted (Fig. 7.28a–e). The fracture healed primarily in a perfect reposition. The patient is free of complaints. The follow-up was documented with the X-rays 14 months after the operation (Fig. 7.28f, g).

Nonunions of the scaphoid are treated with the Herbert's screw; the time to union is reported as between 3 and 14 months (Trumble et al. 1996). With the Diamond TwInS™ procedure, the pseudarthrotic tissue is removed precisely, leaving intact bone which is reinforced by a press-fit bone cylinder from the iliac crest containing bone marrow (Fig. 7.29a–d). The time to union varies between 4 and 6 weeks. Care has being taken to ensure an absolutely stable fracture situation; otherwise, a combination with a screw osteosynthesis is required.

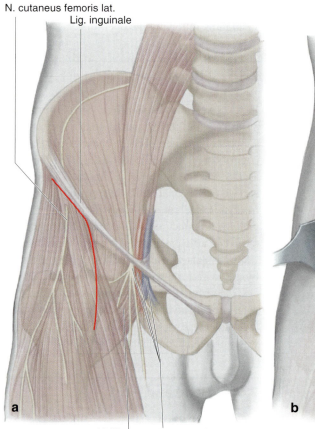
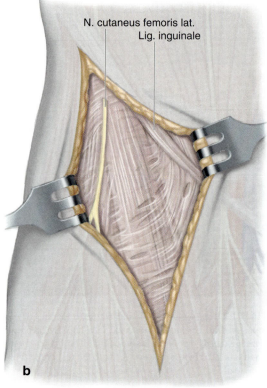
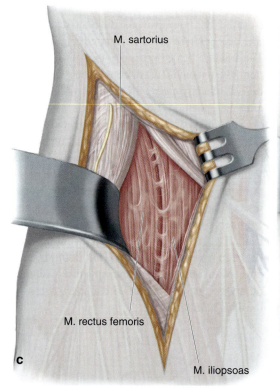
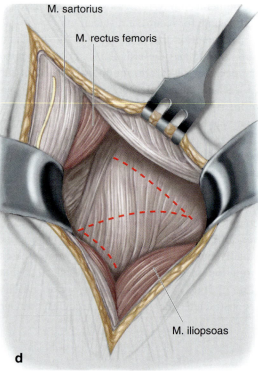

7.6 Hand and Wrist 103

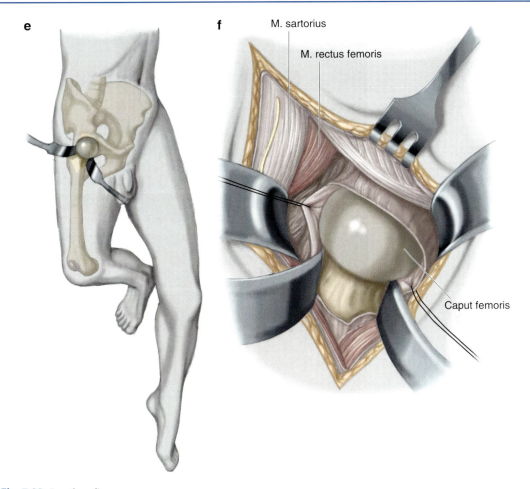

Fig. 7.23 (continued)

Fig. 7.23 (**a–f**) The medial approach according to Draenert preserves all muscles and approaches the joint between the sartorial muscle, the rectus femoris, and the iliopsoas muscle. The heel-strike phase can be exposed by hyperextension of the hip joint (**e, f**). A surgical dislocation is not necessary

Fig. 7.24 (**a–e**) The heel-strike phase can be replaced via the medial approach and hyperextension. The patient has been doing very well for 4 years

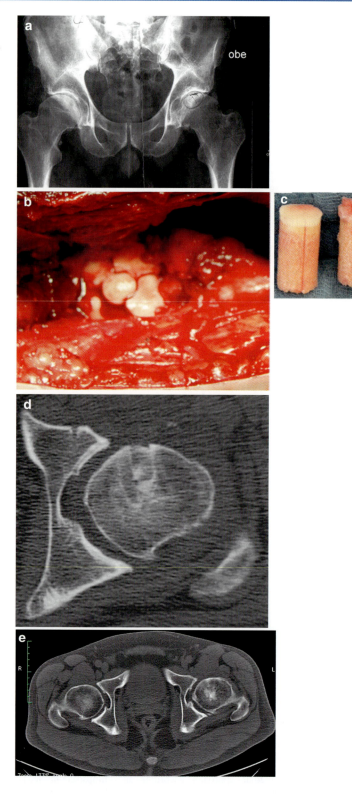

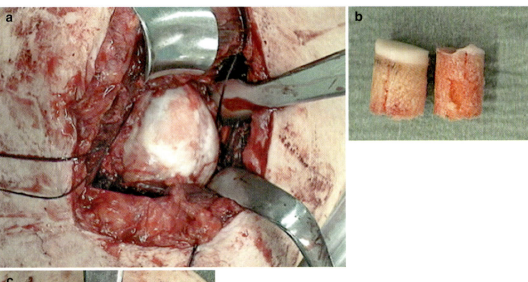
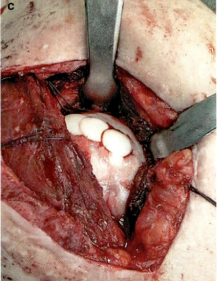

Fig. 7.25 (**a–c**) A reconstruction of an atypical Hill-Sachs's lesion in the shoulder joint has been treated. The patient has remained free of recurrences for 10 years

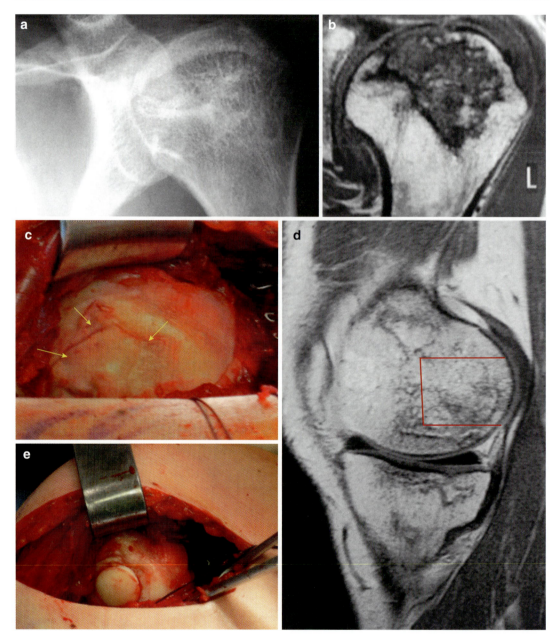

Fig. 7.26 (**a–e**) Necrosis of the humeral head in a 31-year-old man was treated with a graft from the medial distal femoral condyle (**d**). The joint surface was nicely reconstructed. One-and-a-half-year follow-up

7.6 Hand and Wrist

Fig. 7.27 (**a–f**) Transosseous reconstruction of the humero-radial joint in a 42-year-old truck driver yields a perfect result. Four-year follow-up

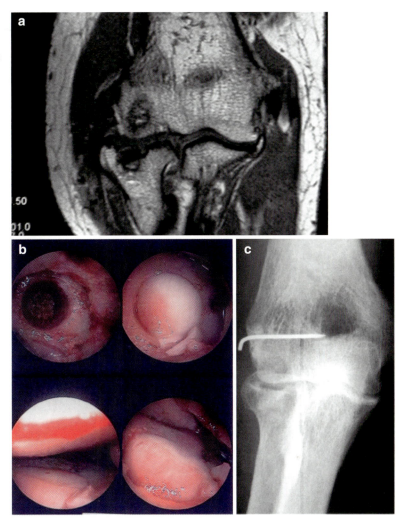

108　　　7　Clinical Practice in Autologous Resurfacing

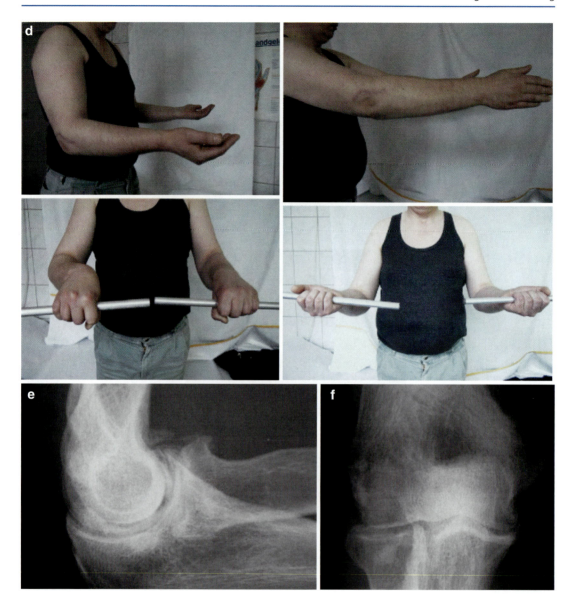

Fig. 7.27 (continued)

Fig. 7.28 (a–g) Reconstruction of a comminuted distal radius fracture in a 42-year-old woman with a perfect result after 1 1/2 years (Erler, Freiberg)

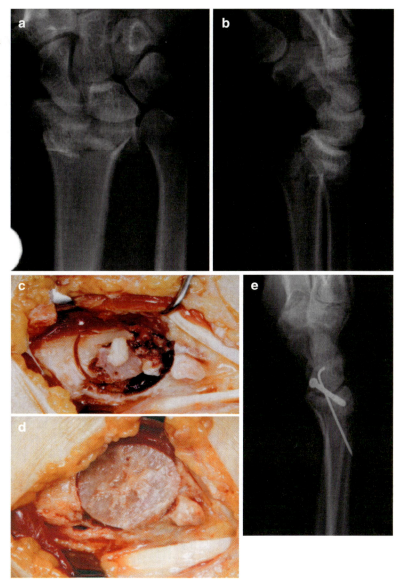

Fig. 7.28 (continued)

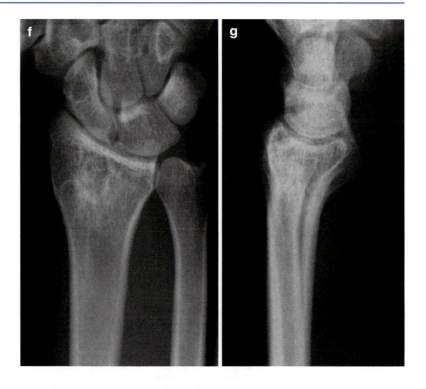

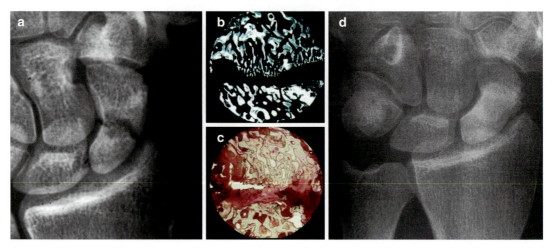

Fig. 7.29 (**a–d**) Nonunion of the scaphoid bone was treated with the Diamond TwInS™ procedure, removing all fibrous tissue of the pseudarthrosis and replacing it with a press-fit graft from the iliac crest: perfect result after 6 weeks. Microradiograph and fuchsine-stained histology of the pseudarthrotic tissue (Paschmeyer, Bremen)

References

Adachi N, Motoyama M, Deie M et al (2009) Histological evaluation of internally-fixed osteochondral lesions of the knee. J Bone Joint Surg 91-B:823–829

Aichroth P (1971) Osteochondral fractures and their relationship to osteochondritis dissecans of the knee. An experimental study in animals. J Bone Joint Surg 53-B:448–455

Bentley G, Biant RW, Carrington M et al (2003) A prospective, randomised comparison of autologous chondrocyte implantation versus mosaicplasty for osteochondral defects in the knee. J Bone Joint Surg 85-B:223–230

Bruns J (1996) Osteochondritis dissecans. Enke, Stuttgart

Diehl K (1976) Zur Biomechanik der intramedullären Prothesenverankerung am coxalen Femurende. Habilitationsschrift. Universität des Saarlandes

Fick R (1904) Handbuch der Anatomie und Mechanik der Gelenke. I.: Anatomie der Gelenke, vol 61. Gustav Fischer, Jena

Fischer O (1903) Der Gang des Menschen. V.Teil: Die Kinematik des Beinschwingens. Anhandl Königl Sächs Ges Wiss 18:23–418

Ganz R, Gill TJ, Gautier E et al (2001) Surgical dislocation of the adult hip. A technique with full access to the femoral head and acetabulum without the risk of avascular necrosis. J Bone Joint Surg 83-B:1119–1124

Gardiner TB (1955) Osteochondritis dissecans in three members of one family. J Bone Joint Surg 37-B:139–141

Gautier E, Ganz K, Krügel N et al (2000) Anatomy of the medial femoral circumflex artery and its surgical implications. J Bone Joint Surg 82-B:679–683

Green WT, Banks HH (1990) Osteochondritis dissecans in children. Clin Orthop Rel Res 255:3–12

König F (1888) Über freie Körper in den Gelenken. Dt Z Chir 27:90–109

Marey (1884) Analyse cinématique de la marche. Comptes rendus 98:1218

Paget J (1870) On the production of some of the loose bodies in joints. St Bartholomew's Hosp Reports 6:1–4

Paré A (1841) Oeuvres complètes, Tome III. JB Baillière, Paris, p 32

Pauwels F (1935) Der Schenkelhalsbruch. Ein mechanisches Problem. Z Orthop Chir 63:1–156

Trumble TE, Clarke T, Kreder HJ (1996) Non-union of the scaphoid. J Bone Joint Surg 78-A:1829–1837

Weber W, Weber E (1836) Mechanik der menschlichen Gehwerkzeuge. In: Merkel F, Fischer O (1894) (eds) Wilhelm Weber's Werk; Kgl. Ges. d. Wiss. Göttingen (Hrg). Springer, Berlin

Yonetani Y, Nakamura N, Natsuume T et al (2010) Histological evaluation of juvenile osteochondritis dissecans of the knee: a case series. Knee Surg Sports Traumatol Arthrosc 18:723–730

Fracture Dowelling

8.1 Osteochondral Fractures

The dowelling of osteocartilage fractures with autologous cartilage-bone dowels using the Diamond TwInS™ technology represents an operative procedure without rival and is considered the method of choice, not only because this procedure avoids a second intervention but moreover because it is the only known procedure which has proven to achieve a restitutio ad integrum. An epiphyseal fragment provides strong epiphyseal cancellous bone and can therefore easily be dowelled using osteocartilage dowels which have also been removed from the epiphysis. There is no alternative as long as the fragment is 6 mm or more thick. A 16-year-old girl was hit by a car while jogging and suffered a posterior dislocation of her right hip with osteocartilage fracture and contusion of the head and fracture of the posterior acetabular rim (Pipkin IV fracture) (Fig. 8.1a, b). The girl was operated on and a free graft, taken from the lower circumference of the head, replaced the severely damaged center of the femoral head; the osteocartilage fragment was refixed with two osteocartilage dowels gathered from the transition zone of the head (Fig. 8.1c). The postoperative follow-up was without complications. The hip healed ad integrum without further interventions. Eighteen years after the operation, the young lady is still actively riding horses and shows no signs of osteoarthritis (Fig. 8.1d, e). A 20-year-old man was injured in a bike accident and suffered a polytrauma, comprising a fracture of the lumbar spine and an osteocartilage fracture of the left hip with a concomitant acetabular rim fracture (Pipkin II) (Fig. 8.2a, b). The patient was operated on using a direct medial approach (Fig. 8.2c) which included "Z"-incision of the capsule and hyperextension of the joint. There was no dislocation necessary. The osteocartilage fragment was too small for refixation and was removed and replaced by a free transplant gathered from the medial distal femoral condyle (Fig. 8.2d–f). The spheroid surface contour of the head was exactly reconstructed. The defect in the posterior condyle was press-fit filled with an HA ceramic (Fig. 8.2g, h).

8.2 Dowelling of Nonunions

Sometimes, there is a last-chance solution to the so-called "hopeless" cases. A 20-year-old woman suffered nonunion of the femoral neck. The bone was already rather atrophic, and the sclerotic fracture line could be considered steep according to Pauwels grade III (Pauwels 1935). The patient had already been marked for a total hip replacement. A 6.5-cm-long bony dowel was gathered from the iliac crest in an orthograde manner, and the lateral femoral cutaneous nerve was not harmed. The dowel was inserted in a cylindrical channel ground by the smaller-sized twin diamond, and the fragments were temporarily fixed with three K-wires (Fig. 8.3a, b). Weight-bearing was allowed beginning with the 13th week. Two

Fig. 8.1 (a–e) Sixteen-year-old girl suffering a Pipkin IV fracture after a car accident. The fragment was dowelled and yielded a perfect result with healing ad integrum (Garde, Iserlohn)

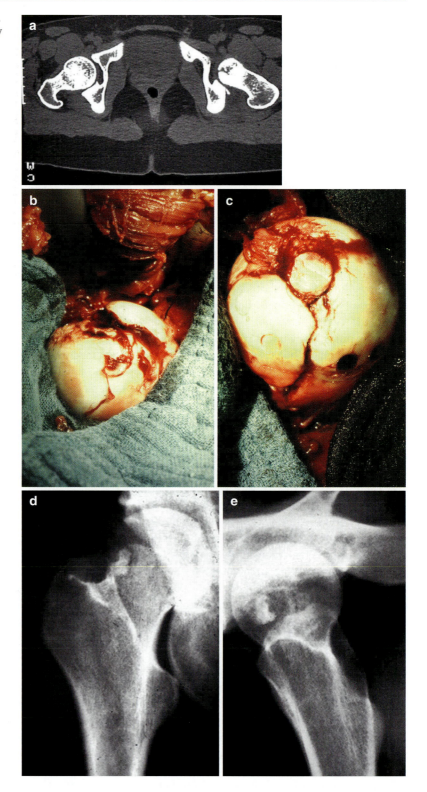

8.2 Dowelling of Nonunions

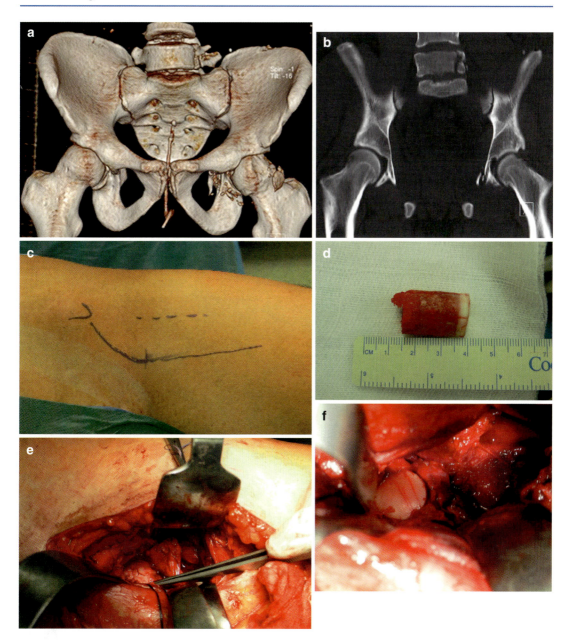

Fig. 8.2 (**a–h**) Pipkin II fracture in a 20-year-old man which was treated with a free graft via a medial approach without dislocation. Perfect result, 2-year follow-up

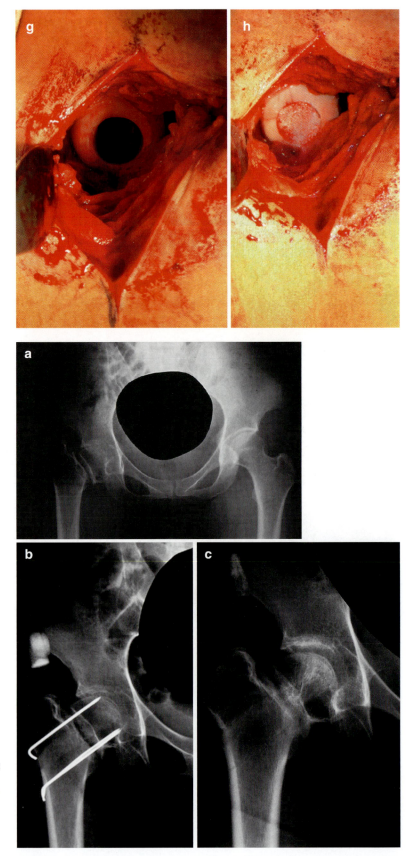

Fig. 8.3 (**a–c**) The dowelling of a nonunion of the femoral neck in a 20-year-old woman yielded a perfect result, thus forming the basis for the recovering of the femoral head. Ten-year follow-up

8.2 Dowelling of Nonunions

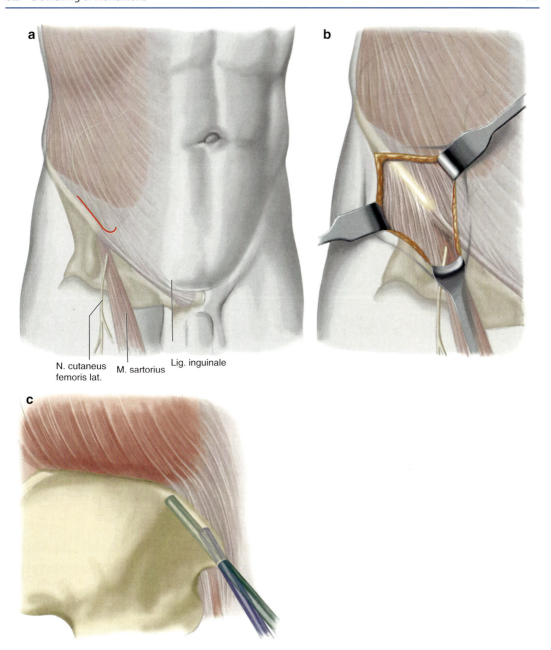

Fig. 8.4 (**a–c**) Anterograde approach to gather long bone cylinders for the dowelling of nonunions. The *blue one* measures 25–35 mm; the *green one* measures 65–75 mm

years after the operation, the young lady jogged, and the hip joint showed free function and a full HS score (Fig. 8.3c). The femoral neck had been reconstructed, and the structure in the femoral head had returned. The follow-up comprises now 10 years. The bony dowel is gathered from the iliac crest in an anterograde manner. The lateral cutaneous femoral nerve has to be prepared (Fig. 8.4a–c).

An 85-year-old lady suffering an infected defect pseudarthrosis of the left femur had been operated on several times and was now confined to bed (Fig. 8.5a, b). There was little hope that she would walk again. The patient was operated on in December: The defect pseudarthrosis was carefully curettaged and finally overbridged by disk grafts taken from the iliac bone, comprising two cortices and bone marrow in between, and the Septopal® chain was removed from the defect (Fig. 8.5c–e). Eight weeks following the operation, the external fixator could be removed, and the patient was walking with the aid of a rollator. In the meantime, the patient is now 87 and is doing very well with crutches. The defect has healed (Fig. 8.5f).

A 42-year-old worker suffering a tibia nonunion was stabilized with a Küntscher's nail following a tibial shaft fracture sustained in a car accident. The fracture did not heal and the nail was finally removed. The patient had already been unable to work for 1½ years. His left tibia was revised and a 75-mm-long corticocancellous

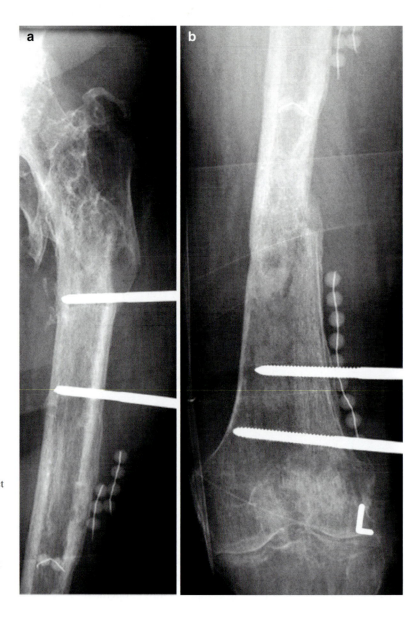

Fig. 8.5 (**a–f**) Infected defect pseudarthrosis in an 85-year-old patient confined to bed. The woman was operated on with disk grafts from the iliac bone and the defect healed (**f**). The patient is now 87 years old and able to walk with crutches

8.2 Dowelling of Nonunions

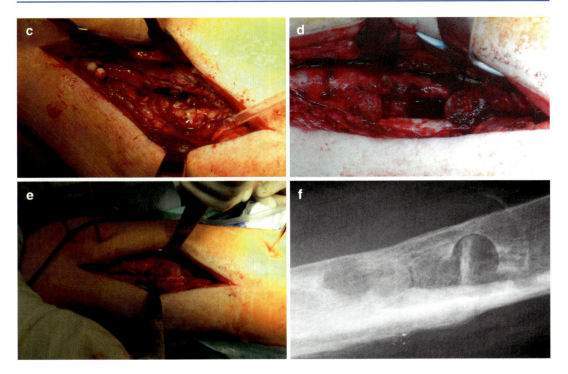

Fig. 8.5 (continued)

bone graft was gathered from the iliac crest. Unfortunately, the lateral femoral cutaneous nerve was damaged during the procedure. The pseudarhtrotic tissue was taken out using diamond twins, and the stable bony dowel was hammered over the pseudarthrotic gap (Fig. 8.6a–c). The nonunion healed without further internal fixation, but a plaster splint was worn for eight weeks. After 3 months, the patient was back in his job.

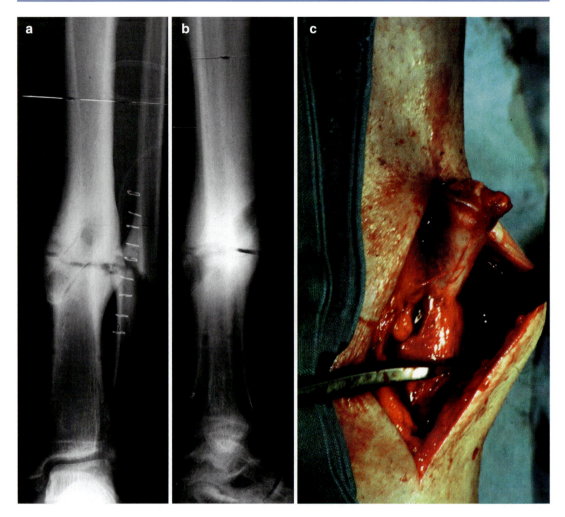

Fig. 8.6 (**a–c**) Dowelled nonunion of the tibia in a 42-year-old man which healed within 8 weeks. The worker is back at his job

Reference

Pauwels F (1935) Der Schenkelhalsbruch. Ein mechanisches Problem. Z Orthop Chir 63:1–156

Bone–Tendon–Bone ACL Plastic

9

The bone–tendon–bone ACL operation with the Diamond TwInS™ technology represents a very elegant procedure. There are five diamond tools necessary. As a first step, the patellar bone-graft cylinder is taken out, together with one-third of the patellar tendon and its bony anchorage with part of the tuberositas patellae. Following the outside-in technique, a transverse cylinder is taken out from the lateral femoral condyle, immediately above the lateral collateral ligament. The patellar tendon is thread through the channel with the bone chip from the tuberositas longitudinally once or twice split, and the bone cylinder is carefully hammered into the lateral femoral condyle. Care has been taken so that the fiber layer below glides over the distal rim of the cylindrical defect. With the K-wire guide, one or – for the double bundle procedure – two cylindrical twin defects are ground with the diamond tool through the tibial head. The patellar tendon is carefully thread through the channel and, since the patellar tendon is longer than the original AC ligament, the fiber bundles of the tendon are sandwich-like pressed by the graft. The graft was taken out from the lateral condyle and is now ground flat on one side, while the bone cylinder is hammered until it appears at the level of the tibial plateau. During the whole process, the tendon is pulled distally over the edge of the tibia. The bony anchorage of the tendon is than carefully sutured to the periosteum of the tibia. As a last step, a bone cylinder is gathered from the iliac crest with the largest of the five diamond tools in an orthograde manner for filling the defect in the patella. Care has to be applied not to damage the lateral femoral cutaneous nerve. The result is an absolutely stable ACL. Rehabilitation can start at least 4 weeks after the intervention (Fig. 9.1a–c). In animal experiments, the bone healing of the double bundle plastic could be shown at the 4-week stage (Fig. 2.17a–e).

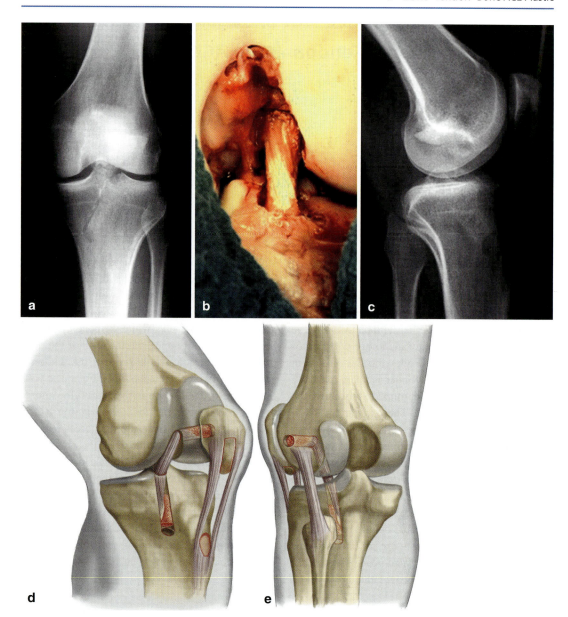

Fig. 9.1 (**a–c**) ACL repair with bone–tendon–bone graft in a 34-year-old man. He started rehabilitation after 6 weeks and has full function. The Diamond TwInS™ technique comprises five diamond tools and is considered very precise and effective. Seven-year follow-up with restitutio ad integrum. (**d, e**) The bone-tendom-bone graft was gathered with the diamond coated tool, and the defect filled with a graft taken out from the iliac crest with the twin-instrument. The diameter of the graft was 1/10 mm larger than the defect in the patella. The bone-tendom-bone graft was pressfit inserted outside-in, immediately above the lateral ligament through the lateral femoral condyle and anchored in the tibial head, where the graft is press-fit fixated with the dowel which has been taken out from the femoral condyle

Instrumentation

10

The surgical Diamond TwInS™ technology evolved in the histological laboratory where bone and mineralized tissue are processed using diamonds and a wet-grinding procedure. The Center of Orthopaedic Sciences (ZOW) in Munich, Germany, has dedicated the last 30 years to developing new technologies to process and photograph macro- and microscopically nondemineralized tissues and to studying bone regeneration, bone healing, and bone remodeling, as well as articular cartilage in three dimensions. Primary bone healing of metaphyseal as well as epiphyseal cancellous bone was studied in animals and human beings. The contact healing of single cancellous bone trabeculae could only be studied by developing a new and very precise technique: the Diamond TwinS technology. It was developed for basic and applied research and, at least in the beginning, not for treatment. The diamond wet-grinding procedure does not traumatize the osteocytes and does not fracture the delicate bone structures. In this way, it was possible to use bone as osteosynthetic material: The bone dowelling technique was born and its bone healing studied in rabbits, dogs, pigs, monkeys, and humans (Draenert and Draenert 1987, 1988). In all cases and indications, the experimental and clinical experience was outstanding, sometimes spectacular; the functional result was perfect; and the healing time was often shorter in comparison to any metallage or artificial implant. It is an outstanding and ongoing experience which might be described as *one step back to biology*.

All sets necessary during the 20 years of experience were carefully composed and, since the precise method does not tolerate any improvisation, all sets have to be available under sterile conditions if a joint reconstruction is started. A piano concert cannot be performed using only one octave.

The short "TM" instruments are the most precise tools.

All three sets are also available as TL versions because the long instruments are necessary for most of the joint reconstructions. The "T" marks the "T"ransplantation, and the thicker walled instruments are marked with "I" = "I"mplantation because they can be used to place artificial implants (Figs. 10.1, 10.2, 10.3, 10.4, 10.5, 10.6, 10.7, 10.8, 10.9, and 10.10).

All six sets are available thicker walled for instrumentation of interventions in compact cortical bone, for fracture treatment, spine operations, nonunions, or metal removal.

The composition of all set is based on 30 years of experience. All sets were essential for one or the other indication to avoid any improvisation. All 13 sets comprise the basic equipment of a transplantation center.

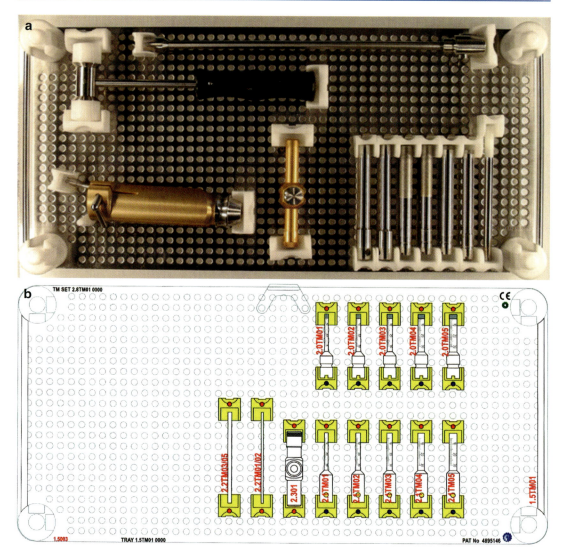

Fig. 10.1 (**a**) Basic instrumentation set; (**b**) biopsy set 2.8 TM 01 comprises delicate transplantation instruments for the dowelling of osteocartilage fragments, biopsies, and hand surgery; (**c**) standard transplantation set 2.8 TM 02 comprises all sizes for the cartilage transplantation; (**d**) large transplantation set 2.8 TM 03 comprises sizes between 17.5 and 21 mm

10 Instrumentation

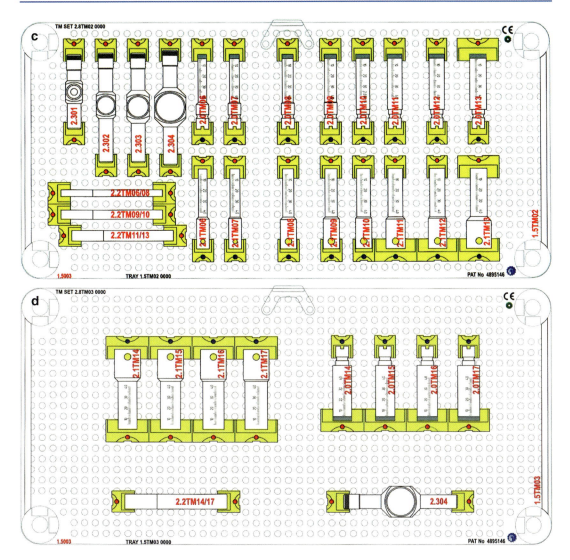

Fig. 10.1 (**c**) Standard, medium sized, transplantation set and (**d**) Transplantation set comprising large diameters

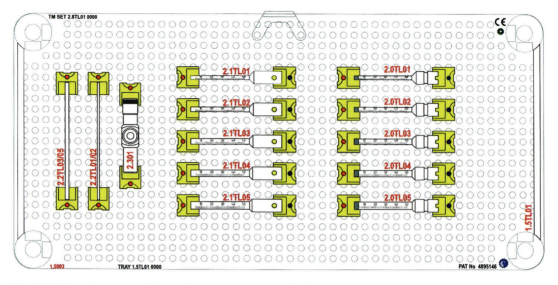

Fig 10.2 Biopsy long set, small transplantation set, necessary for hand surgery, but also for dowelling of cartilage-bone fragments

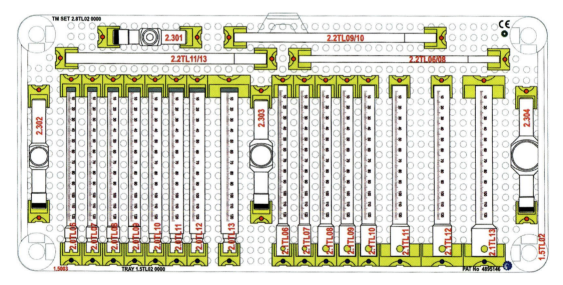

Fig. 10.3 Standard long transplantation set, necessary for bone and ankle reconstruction

10 Instrumentation

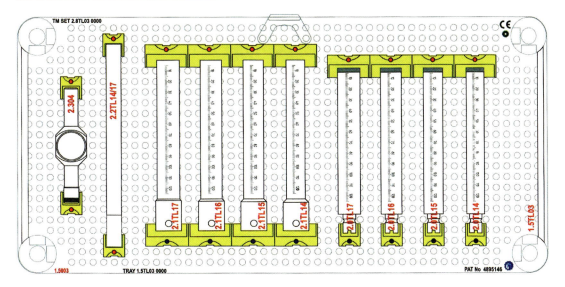

Fig 10.4 Large long transplantation set, necessary for hip and shoulder reconstruction

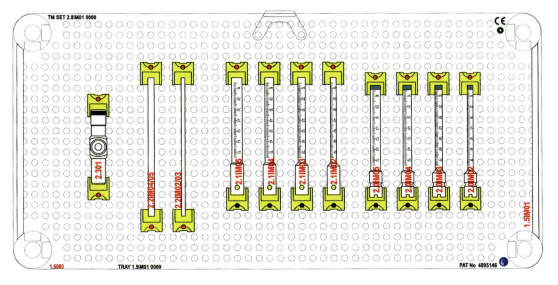

Fig. 10.5 Small implantation set (thicker walled), necessary for ligament refixation, ACL, fracture dowelling, screw removal and other indications

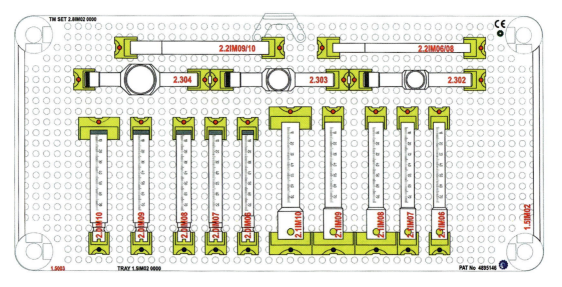

Fig. 10.6 Standard implantation set (thicker walled), necessary for dowelling technique

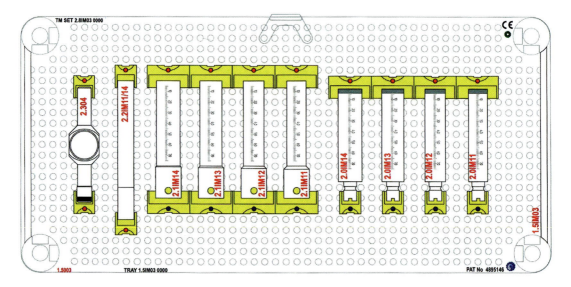

Fig. 10.7 Large implantation set (thicker walled), necessary for all disk graft procedures

10 Instrumentation

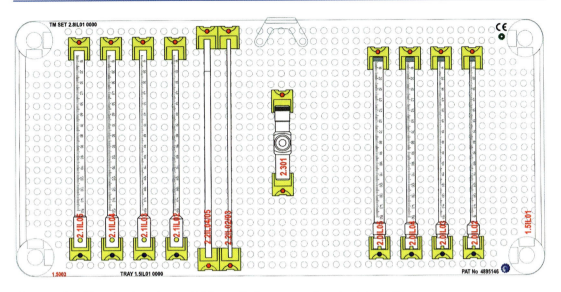

Fig. 10.8 Small long implantation set (thicker walled), necessary for spine interventions

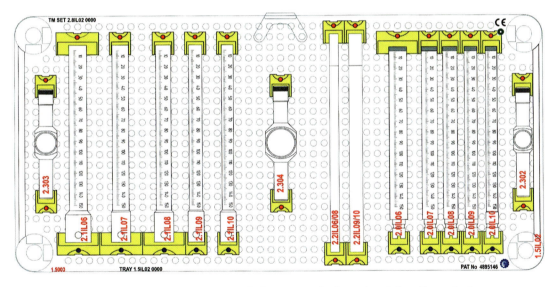

Fig. 10.9 Standard long implantation set (thicker walled), necessary for femoral neck dowelling and spine surgery

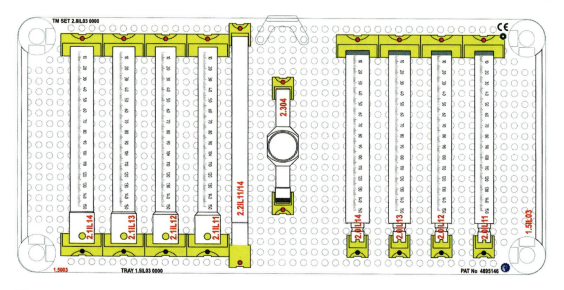

Fig. 10.10 Large long implantation set (thicker walled), necessary for spine surgery and dowelling of nonunions

References

Draenert K and Draenert Y (1987) Ein neues Verfahren für die Knochenbiopsie und die Knorpel-Knochen-Transplantation. Sandorama III:5–12

Draenert K, Draenert Y (1988) A new procedure for bone biopsies and cartilage and bone transplantation. Sandorama III/IV:33–40

Conclusion

11.1 The Success of Autologous Resurfacing and Fracture Dowelling

The success of autologous and even homologous resurfacing is based on the contact healing of the epiphyseal compact and cancellous bone. There is an uninterrupted series of clinical and experimental success (Table 11.1).

The hyaline cartilage represents the gliding coat of the epiphyseal organ, comprising the compact bony baseplate in which all fiber bundles of the cartilage are firmly anchored like the cables of a cable railway. The baseplate transfers the load equally to the elastic cancellous bone. The contact healing of the grafts' and recipients' baseplate conceals the secret of success and discloses why the OATS or mosaicplasty (Hangody et al. 1998) failed: The multiple punches of OATS or mosaicplasty are inserted into drill holes and are reported to heal in contact in the depth of the epiphyseal cancellous bone and not at the level of the compact baseplate, comparable with the picket of a fence.

11.2 The Donor Areals and Defects

Due to the upright position of human beings, two joint compartments reveal a different function compared with four-legged animals: the patellar groove, easily approached, and the posterior face of the femoral condyles. There is a widespread misunderstanding with respect to cancellous bone, which maintains that "cancellous bone heals always." However, a basic fact of research shows that cancellous bone defects actually never heal (Draenert et al. 1981). It is not difficult to be understood. If there is a tube bone, all stresses are convergently transferred to the compact bone tube; if there is, however, a scaffold of bony trabeculae and there is a plate covering them, the load is distributed divergently over all existent trabeculae of the more or less similar stiffness. If some of the trabeculae are missing, the load is carried by the neighboring trabeculae which undergo a lamellar reinforcement. It can thus be concluded that all donor defects have to be carefully filled by a scaffold for osteoconduction, and the gliding surface has to be reconstructed using a pluripotential mesenchymal "cambium" tissue. The best results were achieved with the iliac crest bone comprising two layers of the abdominal muscles, their fibers anchoring in the compact and cancellous bone that contains active bone marrow.

11.3 Osteoconduction by Ceramics

Cancellous bone can be replaced by ceramic bone substitutes. There are different implants available. The bony ingrowth depends upon the specific surface area of the synthetic ceramic implants. Therefore shell-like ceramics show the most pronounced bony ingrowth and form bone-ceramic-bone sandwiches. Shell-like ceramics can be manufactured as hydroxyapatite, as well

Table 11.1 Published work on the transplantation technology

Published work	Key findings	Year
Draenert and Draenert	(Exp) prim.metaph.bone healing	1979
Draenert and Draenert	(Exp) gap healing of compact bone	1980
Draenert et al.	(Exp) contact healing of metaphyseal bone; (clin) contact healing of dowels: nonunion of the fem. neck and tibia; FH necroses	1981
Draenert	(Exp) prim. bone healing of autologous and homologous grafts	1982
Draenert	(Exp, clin) metaph. bone healing	1983
Draenert and Draenert	(Exp) epiph. bone healing; the diamond concept	1987/1988 (E)
Rischke et al.	(Clin) biological treatment of osteoarthritis of the knee	1997
Laprell and Petersen	(Clin) osteochondral grafts knee – 4–14-year results	2001
Hochstein et al.	(Clin) autologous resurfacing	2001
Slodicka et al.	(Clin) scaphoid grafting with SDI	2002
Draenert et al.	(Exp, clin) la guarigione primaria della cartilagine e dell'osso spugnoso	2002
Draenert et al.	(Exp) histology of different drills	2007

as β-TCP implants. The latter will be of advantage in or near the joint and for children; hydroxyapatite, which is stiffer and nearly not reabsorbable, is advantageously applied in defects under load or exposed to stresses. Both implants are suitable to fill donor defects in a press-fit-like manner. On the other hand, it is a fact, proven by applied research, that the bone-forming element is a bead. Primary formation of cancellous bone will take place around ceramic beads which cannot, however, act as a press-fit implant (Draenert et al. 2011). Donor defects filled with ceramics in a press-fit-like manner resist to stresses acting upon the defect and do not give rise to donor bed morbidity (Draenert et al. 2001).

References

Draenert K (1982) Stabil implantiertes auto-und homologes Spongiosatransplantat. In: Hackenbroch MH, Refior HJ, Jäger M (eds) Osteogenese und Knochenwachstum. Georg Thieme, Stuttgart, pp 177–184

Draenert K (1983) Beobachtungen über die metaphysäre Knochenheilung. In: Rütt A, Küsswetter W (eds) Gelenknahe Osteotomien bei der Dysplasiehüfte des Adoleszenten und jungen Erwachsenen. Georg Thieme, Stuttgart, pp 4–15

Draenert K, Draenert Y (1979) The architecture of metaphyseal bone healing. SEM. SEM Inc., O'Hare, pp 521–528

Draenert K, Draenert Y (1980) Gap healing of compact bone. Scanning electron microscope II, pp 57–71

Draenert Y, Draenert K (1981) Histo-Morphologie der Tangentialfaserschicht nach Kreuzbandläsion. Eine tierexperimentelle Studie am Kniegelenk der Ratte. In: Jäger M, Hackenbroch MH, Refior HJ (Hrg) (eds) Kapselbandläsionen des Kniegelenkes. Georg Thieme, Stuttgart, pp S.88–S.92

Draenert K, Draenert Y (1987) Ein neues Verfahren für die Knochenbiopsie und die Knorpel-Knochen-Transplantation. Sandorama III:5–12

Draenert K, Draenert Y (1988) A new procedure on bone biopsies and cartilage and bone transplantation. Sandorama III/IV, pp 33–40

Draenert K, Draenert Y, Springorum HW et al (1981) Histo-Morphologie des Spongiosadefektes und die Heilung des autologen Spongiosatransplantates. In: Cotta H, Martini AK (Hrg) (eds) Implantate und Transplantate in der Plastischen und Wiederherstellungschirurgie. Springer, Berlin

Draenert K, Wiese FG, Garde U et al (2001) Synthetische Knochenersatzwerkstoffe auf HA- und TCP-Basis. Trauma Berufskrankh 4:293–300

Draenert K, Draenert Y, Bombelli R et al (2002) La guarigione primaria della cartilagine e dell'osso spugnoso ed il suo significato clinico. GIOT 28:531–539

Draenert FG, Mathys R Jr, Ehrenfeld M et al (2007) Histological examination of drill sites in bovine rib bone after in vitro with eight different devices. BJ Oral Maxillofac Surg 45:548–552

Draenert K, Draenert M, Erler M et al (2011) How bone forms in large cancellous defects: critical analysis based on experimental work and literature. Injury, Int J Care Injured 42:47–55

Hangody L, Kish G, Karpati Z et al (1998) Mosaicplasty for the treatment of articular cartilage defects: application in clinical practice. Orthopedics 21:751–756

References

Hochstein P, Schmickal T, Wentzensen A (2001) Autologes Resurfacing der Gelenkoberfläche. Trauma Berufskrankh Suppl 3:5365–5369

Laprell H, Petersen W (2001) Autologous osteochondral transplantation using the diamond bone-cutting system (DBCS): 6–12 years' follow-up of 35 patients with osteochondral defects at the knee joint. Arch Orthop Trauma Surg 121:248–253

Rischke B, Garde U, Draenert K et al (1997) Biologische Gelenksanierung bei Gonarthrose mit Knorpel-Knochen-Dübeln. Extracta Orthop 11:12–15

Slodicka R, Regel G, Draenert K (2002) Die Zylinderfrästechnik (Surgical Diamond Initiative - SDI) für Therapie der Kahnbeinpseudarthrose. Akt Traumatol 32:278–282

Subject Index

A
α-Whitlockit structure, 44
Anisotropic structure, 41
Ankle joint and foot, 87–92
Autologous, 131

B
β-tricalcium phosphate, 41
β-Whitlockit structure, 44
Biodegradation, 46–48
Bioglasses, 41
BMP 2, 36
BMP 7, 36
Bone–ceramic–bone sandwich, 42
Bone dowelling technique, 123
Bone dowels, 67–68
Bone–tendon–bone ACL, 121
Bony baseplate, 61

C
Cambium layer, 87
Cancellous bone healing, 36
Cartilage-bone cylinders, 60
Ceramic disease, 49
Ceramic reinforced bone, 46
Chondral, 31
Chondroitin, 3
Chondroitin sulfate, 3
Cold stage, 14
Compressive strength, 41
Conductive ladder, 48
Continuous passive motion, 84
Conversion to compact bone, 34
Coralliform calcium carbonate, 42
Craquelé fractures, 81, 84
Cruciate ligaments, 31

D
Damping properties, 49
Degradation process, 46
Diamond-coated instruments, 53
TwInS™ Diamond twins, 55, 61, 92
Diamond twinS" technology, 123

E
Disk grafts, 118
Donor bed, 71
Donor defects, 87
Dowelling of osteocartilage fractures, 113
Dowels, 61

E
Elbow, 101
Extraction procedure, 54
Extractor, 54

F
Fissures, 81
Flip osteotomy, 92
Foot-to-ground phase, 94
Fractures, 31

G
Growth plate, 21

H
HA implant, 87
Hand and wrist, 101–111
Heel-strike osteoarthritis, 94–101
Heel-strike phase, 92, 94
Hill-Sachs, 100
Homologous cartilage-bone grafts, 31
Human osteogeny, 1, 3
Hydroxyapatite, 41, 84

I
ICDD. *See* International Center for Diffraction Data (ICDD)
Iliac crest, 63
Infected defect pseudarthrosis, 118
International Center for Diffraction Data (ICDD), 44

J
JCPDS standards, 44

L
Lamellar reinforcement, 34
Lamina splendens, 3
Large cartilage, 77
Lavage system, 68

M
Macrophagocytes, 46
Microcrystals, 43
Morbidity of the iliac crest, 63
Morsellized cancellous bone, 48
Multinuclear giant cells, 46

O
OATS or mosaicplasty, 131
Observationes anatomicae, 1
Osseointegration, 45
Osseous drift, 24
Osteoarthritis, 81
Osteocartilage dowels, 113
Osteocartilage fractures, 68–71
Osteochondral fractures, 31
Osteochondral fragment, 67
Osteochondritis dissecans, 81, 87–92
Osteoconductive scaffolds, 48
Osteointegration, 45
Osteologia Nova, 4, 10
Osteosyntheses of the pelvis, 92

P
Patellar groove, 66, 71
Patellar tendon, 121
Pestle, 61
Pipkin IV fracture, 113
Pluripotential mesenchymal cells, 87

R
Rearthroscopies, 66
Remodeling, 34, 47
Replaminiform process, 42
Resorption, 47
Resurfacing, 131

S
Scanning electron microscope, 14
Septopal® chain, 118
Shell bone, 42
Shoulder, 100–101
Silberberg mouse, 29
Synthacer®, 46, 84, 87
Syntricer®, 46

T
Talus, 87
"Toe-off" phase, 94
Traumatic osteocartilage defects, 77
Triple graft, 64
Twin diamond dowelling technique, 67
Twin instruments, 57
TwInS™, 101

U
Ultrasonic bath, 56

W
Wet-grinding instruments, 59
Wet-grinding procedure, 53
Woven bone, 34

X
X-ray diffractometry, 44

Author Index

A
Adachi, N., 81
Agholme, F., 36
Ahlers, J., 31
Aichroth, P., 81
Alberty-Ryoppy, A., 32
Albinus, B.S., 4
Allen, T., 41
Altmann, K., 34
Ameil, M., 32
Andrades, J.A., 13
Andreassen, T.T., 31
Andrews, J.R., 31
Angermann, P., 32
Axhausen, G., 34

B
Bachelin, P., 31
Balzsy, J.E., 31
Banks, H.H., 81
Barber, F.A., 31
Barnett, C.H., 13
Bassett, F.H., 31
Baudenbacher, R., 32
Bauer, T.W., 41
Beaufils, P., 16, 31
Becerra, J., 13
Belchier, J., 8
Bellaiche, L., 31
Benedetto, K.P., 32
Benninghoff, A., 2
Bentley, G., 81
Berndt, A.L., 31
Bernier, J.M., 32
Biant, R.W., 81
Biedermann, W., 4
Blasier, R.B., 31
Bloom, W., 23
Bohart, P.G., 31
Boitzy, A., 34
Bomberg, B.C., 31
Bosse, M.J., 31
Boszotta, H., 31
Bruns, J., 81
Bugmann, P., 31

Bunker, T.D., 32
Buring, K., 34
Burkhardt, R., 53
Burkus, J.K., 31
Butler, J.C., 31

C
Cameron, C.H.S., 13
Canale, S.T., 31
Carrington, M., 81
Chan, S.M., 13
Charnley, J., 34
Cheselden, W., 1
Clarke, I.C., 13
Clarke, T., 101
Cochrane, W., 13
Cohen, P., 31
Cordey, J., 34
Culman, K., 4

D
Dahmen, G., 32
Danckwardt-Lilliestrom,
   G., 31
Danis, R., 34
Dantschakoff, W., 21
Davies, V.D., 13
Deie, M., 81
Dell'accio, F., 29
Detlie, T., 31
Deutsch, A.L., 31
Deutsch, C., 4
Diehl, K., 94
Dobyns, J.H., 31
Draenert, A.I., 42
Draenert, F.G., 53
Draenert, K., 34, 53, 123, 131, 132
Draenert, M., 132
Draenert, Y., 13, 34, 53, 123, 131
Du Hamel, H.L., 8, 32
Duparc, F., 16
Dupuytren, G., 32
Duraine, G., 13
Dutkowsky, J., 31, 32

E
Edson, D.M., 31
Ehrenfeld, M., 53
Enlow, D.H., 21
Erler, M., 132

F
Fallopius, G., 1
Feder, K.S., 31
Fick, R., 77
Fischer, O., 94
Flourens, P., 10
Foster, B.K., 31, 32
Fowler, P.J., 31
Frank, A., 31
Frankl, U., 31
Freeman, B.L., 31, 32
Frenkel, S.R., 29
Fu, F., 31

G
Galilei, G., 4
Ganz, K., 17, 92
Ganz, R., 17, 92, 94
Garde, U., 68, 132
Gardiner, T.B., 81
Gardner, D.L., 13
Garrett, W.E. Jr, 31
Gautier, E., 17, 92, 94
Gegenbaur, C., 4
Gelbermann, R.H., 31
Gelman, M.I., 31
Gerard, Y., 32
Gerber, F., 19
Ghadially, F.N., 13
Gilbert, T.J., 31
Gilley, J.S., 31
Gill, T.J., 17, 92, 94
Glotzer, W., 32
Green, D.P., 31
Green, W.T., 81
Grogan, S.P., 31
Gross, A.E., 32
Guerado, E., 13

H
Haddad, R.J., 31
Hales, S., 8
Hammar, S.A., 2
Hämmerle, C.P., 31
Hamze, B., 31
Hangody, L., 131
Hannouche, D., 16
Hardaker, W.J. Jr, 31
Harilainen, A., 32
Harty, M., 30

Harvell, J.C., 31
Harvey, W., 4
Havers, C., 4
Hayward, I., 32
Heidenhain, R., 2
Hellmann, W., 13
Hench, L.L., 41
Herron, M., 32
Holmes, R.E., 42
Holzheimer, R., 31
Hontas, M.J., 31
Hou, X.K., 29
Howship, J., 4
Hultkrantz, W., 2
Huylebroek, J.F., 31

I
Imai, Y., 29
Isaacs, C.L., 31
Isaksson, H., 36

J
Jacob, R.P., 31
Johnson, E., 31
Jones, P., 31
Joyce, F., 31

K
Karlsson, C., 31
Karpati, Z., 131
Keller, J., 31
Kember, N.F., 23
Kenny, C.H., 31
Khasawneh, Z.M., 32
Kish, G., 131
Kleinschmidt, A.K., 13
Kölliker, R., 4
König, F., 34, 81
Korn, U., 32
Kreder, H.J., 101
Kristensen, G., 32
Krompecher, St., 34
Krügel, N., 17, 92
Kuang, Y., 29
Kunze, K., 31
Kusnick, C., 32
Kuusela, T., 32

L
Lane, W.A., 34
Lange, F., 68
Laredo, J.D., 31
Larson, B., 31
Lavard, P., 32
Lemnius, L., 8

Author Index

Lewis, P.L., 31, 32
Lexer, E., 34, 68
Lieberkühn, N., 4
Light, T.R., 31
Lindahl, A., 31
Lind, T., 32
Li, X., 36
Longmore, R.B., 13
Lorenz, H., 32
Lubarsch, O., 34
Lutten, C., 32

M

MacConnail, M.A., 3
Maquire, J.K., 31
Marey, E.-J., 94
Marks, P.H., 31
Maroudas, A., 13
Martens, M., 31
Mathys, R. Jr., 53
Matzen, P.F., 34
Maximow, A., 21
Mazel, C., 31
McElfresh, E.C., 31
McGinty, J.B., 31
McKee, N.H., 32
McLean, F.C., 23
McNamee, P.B., 32
Mehrara, B.J., 29
Meiss, L., 47, 49
Meyers, M.H., 32
Miligram, J.W., 31
Mink, J.H., 31
Miyaki, S., 31
Mizaldus, A., 8
Mjoberg, B., 31
Mooar, L.A., 31
Morrey, B.F., 31
Morris, V.B., 31
Motoyama, M., 81
Müller, H., 8
Myllynen, P., 32

N

Nakamura, N., 81
Natsuume, T., 81
Nesbitt, R., 1
Neu, C.P., 13
Noyes, F.R., 31

O

O'Brien, E.T., 31
Ogden, J.A., 31
Otsuki, S., 31
Ove, P.N., 31

P

Paar, O., 31
Padovani, J.P., 31
Paget, J., 81
Pais, M.J., 31
Paré, A., 81
Parisien, J.S., 31
Paulos, L., 31
Pauwels, F., 34, 94, 113
Pavlov, H., 31
Perren, S.M., 34
Pettine, K.A., 31
Phemister, D.B., 68
Pritzker, K.P., 32
Prudich, J.F., 31

Q

Quintin, A., 31

R

Rae, P.S., 32
Ragnarsson, B., 32
Ranvier, L., 15, 21
Redl, H., 32
Rees, W., 32
Reinert, C.M., 31
Ricklin, P., 32
Riegels-Nielsen, P., 32
Rigault, P., 31
Robin, C., 4
Rosenberg, L., 13
Roy, S., 13
Runow, A., 31

S

Saadeh, P.B., 29
Saffar, P., 31
Sartoris, D.J., 32
Scaletta, C., 31
Schaffer, J., 2
Schenk, R., 34
Schild, H., 31
Schizas, C., 31
Schlag, G., 32
Schlesinger, L.C., 31
Schleyden, M., 4
Schmiedeberg, O., 3
Schonholtz, G.J., 31
Schreiber, F.C., 31
Schwann, T., 4
Scott, T.D., 32
Scranton, P.E. Jr., 31
Shors, E.C., 42
Silverman, B.F., 34
Simon, J.P., 31
Smith, S.T., 41

Sperner, G., 32
Splinter, R.J., 41
Springorum, H.W., 53
Stanitski, C.L., 31
Stripling, W.D., 31
Sun, J., 29

T
Talke, M., 31, 32
Tehranzadeh, J., 31
Thomas, W., 32
Thompson, S.K., 32
Tokuhara, Y., 29
Torg, J.S., 31
Trumble, T.E., 101

U
Urist, M.R., 34

V
Vanarthos, W., 31
Vandell, R.F., 31
Vangsness, T., 31
van Leeuwenhoek, A., 4
Vellet, A.D., 31
Venn, M., 13
Vesalius, A., 1
Vincent, T.L., 29
Virchow, R., 4

Visuri, T., 32
Voetsch, A., 34
von Meyer, H., 4

W
Wagner, H., 34
Wakintani, S., 29
Wardrop, R.W., 42
Wasilewski, S.A., 31
Weber, F., 94
Weber, J.N., 42
Weber, W., 94
Weh, L., 32
Weidenreich, F., 4, 17, 42
Wertheimer, S.J., 31
White, E., 42
White, N.W., 42
White, R.A., 42
Wiese, F.G., 132
Willenegger, H., 34
Wilson, W.J., 31
Wolff, J., 4
Wolford, L.M., 42
Wurmbach, H., 34

Y
Yonetani, Y., 81

Z
Zilch, H., 31, 32